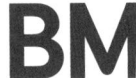

BMA Li**
Better know
Information p

By borrowing
1. The item
   details b
2. The item
3. Long-ter
   required
4. PROO

James Woollard and Josie Jenkinson

RCPsych Publications

 BRITISH MEDICAL ASSOCIATION

© The Royal College of Psychiatrists 2016

RCPsych Publications is an imprint of the Royal College of Psychiatrists,
21 Prescot Street, London E1 8BB
http://www.rcpsych.ac.uk

All rights reserved. No part of this book may be reprinted or reproduced or utilised in any form or by any electronic, mechanical, or other means, now known or hereafter invented, including photocopying and recording, or in any information storage or retrieval system, without permission in writing from the publishers.

British Library Cataloguing-in-Publication Data.
A catalogue record for this book is available from the British Library.
ISBN 978-1-909726-54-3

Distributed in North America by Publishers Storage and Shipping Company.

The views presented in this book do not necessarily reflect those of the Royal College of Psychiatrists, and the publishers are not responsible for any error of omission or fact.

The Royal College of Psychiatrists is a charity registered in England and Wales (228636) and in Scotland (SC038369).

Printed by Bell & Bain Limited, Glasgow, UK.

Contents

Abbreviations		iv
Preface		v
Introduction		vi

Part 1. Core skills

1	Core communication skills	3
2	Verbal communication skills	12
3	Taking control	19
4	Structured presentations	27
5	Physical examination, investigations and cognitive assessment	30

Part 2. Planning your preparation

6	Developing the right knowledge	37
7	Individual preparation	39
8	Group preparation	43
9	The day of the exam	45

Part 3. Putting skills into practice – mock stations

10	Mock session 1: Finding your voice	49
11	Mock session 2: Talking techniques	53
12	Mock session 3: Taking control	57
13	Mock session 4: Structured stations	61

Resources	63
Appendix	65
Index	69

Abbreviations

A&E	accident and emergency department
ADHD	attention-deficit hyperactivity disorder
AIMS	Abnormal and Involuntary Movements Scale
CASC	Clinical Assessment of Skills and Competencies
CAT	cognitive analytic therapy
CBT	cognitive–behavioural therapy
ECG	electrocardiogram
EPSE	extrapyramidal side-effects
GP	general practitioner
MMSE	Mini Mental State Examination
NHS	National Health Service
NICE	National Institute for Health and Care Excellence
NLP	neurolinguistic programming
OSCE	Objective Structured Clinical Examination

Preface

A shared view of our colleagues who have passed the Clinical Assessment of Skills and Competencies (CASC) exam – the final membership exam of the Royal College of Psychiatrists – is that our day-to-day clinical practice should have gone a long way in preparing us for it. We also felt that the preparation for the exam and the intense reflective learning we undertook as a part of that made us all better clinicians. The first and most important message of this book is that practice for the CASC should begin on day 1 of your training in psychiatry so that when you come to take the exam, although a significant hurdle, you are able to see it as an opportunity to display the subtle and refined skills you have developed over the years. In our experience, real life is far more challenging than the controlled environment of the CASC.

An ability to adapt the qualities of your voice, body language, questioning technique and structure under pressure is one of the keys to passing the CASC and will help you develop into an excellent clinician. We expect that you are already using this ability, perhaps unknowingly, as a part of your everyday communication. If you are not aware you are doing this, then recognition is the first step. Mastering this ability will take preparation, whether by reviewing videos of your performance or following verbal and written feedback after mock stations. Taking the approach of realistic, honest and open self-reflection with a preparedness to challenge yourself is an important part of your preparation. We hope that this book will act as a guide for this approach.

Introduction

Background

We are assuming that if you are reading this you are planning to sit the Clinical Assessment of Skills and Competencies (CASC) exam of the Royal College of Psychiatrists at some point in the future. It may be that you are currently in a training post either in or outside the UK, or working in a non-training post in psychiatry. Of course it may also be that you have interest in developing the skills required for the exam in those that you supervise or mentor.

As such, some of you may already know the details of the exam and perhaps have even sat it before. For those who are new to the exam, we will start by outlining the basics.

The CASC exam

The CASC exam has been the final membership examination of the Royal College of Psychiatrists since 2008. In its current form the exam involves two circuits of eight 'stations'. The examination is held over the course of 1 day, with a morning and afternoon session. The morning circuit involves four paired stations of 10 min each with 90 s of reading time before each station. The afternoon circuit involves eight stand-alone stations, again with 90 s of reading time before each station.

For paired stations, information gathered in the first station is used in the following one, for example taking a history from a patient in the first station and discussing the assessment with their relative in the second.

Currently, to be eligible to sit the exam you need to have passed all written papers set by the College and have 24 months of whole-time equivalent post-foundation or internship experience in psychiatry. Detailed and up-to-date eligibility criteria can be found on the examination pages of the College's website, www.rcpsych.ac.uk/traininpsychiatry/examinations.aspx

INTRODUCTION

Structure of this book and how to use it

This book has three main sections. Part 1 describes core verbal and non-verbal communication skills, and outlines techniques for their development and practice. There are also techniques for managing time, taking control, as well as when and how to use a more structured approach. This section concludes with a chapter on the specific procedural skills that are tested in the exam, such as physical examination, cognitive assessment and interpretation of investigations.

Part 2 moves on to consider how best to prepare for the exam, both as an individual and in a group. It describes how to develop your knowledge base and organise your group practice, and gives specific advice for the actual day of the exam.

Part 3 is a collection of mock stations. These have been specifically developed to match the skills and techniques outlined in Part 1, and ideally should be used in conjunction with the relevant chapters. Throughout the text we will identify the mock stations relevant to the skills being discussed. Mock stations will also start with the key skills required as an aide-memoire. As such you could either work through this book in order, practising the stations as they arise, or you could read Parts 1 and 2 straight through and then practise the stations in any order, referring back to the relevant section to remind yourself of the details of each technique as necessary.

Person-centred approach

Although we recognise that there are different approaches to the practice of psychiatry across the world, this book has been written with the person-centred approach at its core. This is reflective of the current ideals of clinical care within the National Health Service (NHS).

Being person-centred means (The Health Foundation, 2014):

- affording people dignity, respect and compassion
- offering coordinated care, support or treatment
- offering personalised care, support or treatment
- being enabling – helping people to help themselves.

If this approach is new to you, then we would suggest you spend some time familiarising yourself with the four principles above. When practising the skills outlined in this book, consider how this approach could be reflected in the language and style of communication you develop.

Adaptation

In your early practice, focusing on each of the different chapters in turn will help you fully develop the skills within them. Do not punish yourself if you

vii

are trying to practise one skill and completely mess up another in a mock station or assessment. Over time you will become more competent in each skill and eventually that skill will partly pass into unconscious processing. In this way you will begin 'automatically' to build rapport and structure in all your contact with patients.

Depending on your ability already, and the intensity with which you are going to practise these techniques, you will need to spend a good 6 months in preparation before the exam. Over time the skills will become incorporated into your everyday work and by the time you get to the exam they will flow naturally.

We can only encourage you to be playful and not be afraid to appear foolish when practising these techniques. Through this openness of experience, you will quickly learn how to use these techniques for yourself, in your own natural style.

Although not essential, it is helpful to try to develop a 'third umpire' (to use a cricketing term) when practising for the CASC. The third umpire is that part of your conscious awareness that sits at the sidelines and monitors what is going on between you and the patient in real time. This umpire gives you the feedback you need to adapt your style or technique in the station. Being able to use this metacognitive umpire takes practice and should be initially developed in comfortable situations (such as conversations with friends) when it will not matter if you lose track of what is going on.

Many of the people we have met in preparing for the CASC appeared to be trying to learn a script for every possible station that may exist. For us this is akin to learning a script for every patient interaction that you may ever have. Not only is this obviously impossible but it also suggests a limited ability to deal with evolving human interactions. If you have been learning scripts in anticipation of a set outcome, then not only are you setting yourself a very difficult memory test of remembering all the stations, but you are also giving yourself false reassurance. As soon as a station deviates from the script you have learned, you will be left in a heightened state of anxiety, which will inevitably impair your performance. We cannot emphasise enough that learning scripts for each station is not the way to pass the exam.

If you have been preparing by trying to learn scripts for each station, then try asking yourself this question: what worry stops me from trusting my ability to work with whatever scenario I am faced with? Tackling the answer to this question may be difficult, but it is worth bearing in mind that we expect our patients to answer equally difficult questions of themselves every day.

Reference

The Health Foundation (2014) *Person-Centred Care Made Simple: What Everyone Should Know about Person-Centred Care*. The Health Foundation.

Part 1

Core skills

CHAPTER 1

Core communication skills

In this first chapter, we are going to focus on the foundations of your performance in the CASC exam, however the skills outlined here should not just be restricted to preparing for the exams, as they form the basis of effective communication with anyone.

You may in fact be using some or all of these techniques already without realising it. They appear relatively simple, but mastering them can be difficult as this requires a conscious monitoring of your own body posture, tone of voice and choice of phrase or words; all of which can feel awkward and uncomfortable at first.

These techniques require practice. To allow them to become as natural as possible, you should not just practise them in clinical settings but play with them in every interaction. As when learning any new skill, there is a transition from unconscious incompetence, through the awkward phase of conscious incompetence (where it might seem like every word you choose seems forced), to a phase of conscious competence. With time, the aim is to develop unconscious competence, at which point these techniques will be at their most powerful (Howell, 1982). So why are these techniques important? They work on an unconscious level to affect how others perceive the quality of your communication and interactions. This is not only true of the patient or actor you are talking to, but also of the examiner observing you. Done well, no one will notice them unless they are specifically looking out for them; but an observer is likely to see that rapport is established rapidly between the doctor and the patient and that communication is sympathetic and fluid.

Time to act: recognising different aspects of communication

The CASC can be seen as a series of performances and, as such, taking on the behaviours of a performing actor can help. Throughout their training, actors learn to use their voices and become comfortable with the ranges and variations they may effect. To use the techniques outlined on the following pages it is useful to begin to get a sense of how you may vary your voice.

You will need to know how to use these variations to deploy skilfully non-verbal communication.

As a part of your early CASC training, play with your voice. Shout loudly, talk quietly, try different inflections at the beginning and end of sentences. Record your voice and listen to it, getting to know your inflections and any vocal tics you might have. Think about developing a consultation voice – professional while conveying an innate sense of empathy through its tone and character.

There is an observation that a rising inflection at the end of sentence, as in the caricature of an Australian accent, implies a questioning statement. A descending tone at the end of sentence implies a more commanding statement. This subtle change in tone within a sentence is the kind of moment-by-moment change you should become comfortable with. You may be making these changes naturally and in becoming aware of them, you may become awkward and clumsy. With increasing awareness, you will be able to use these changes more purposefully.

A key exercise here is to listen to other people's speech qualities. Using that metacognitive third umpire, 'listen in' to how someone changes their voice during their sentences and over the course of a conversation. Then listen in to yourself and observe the changes in your own voice. How is it different to others? If you hear a voice you like, what is it about that voice that appeals to you?

Vocal warm-ups

Here are some vocal warm-ups to get you going and using your voice to its full potential. Do not be embarrassed!

Pumpkin face/Raisin face

This is saying 'Pumpkin face!', making your whole face as big as a pumpkin (with a voice to match), and then screwing your face up as small as a raisin while saying 'Raisin face!' in a tiny screwed up voice.

Vowel punching

You can go through vowel sounds while punching the air in front of you to make the sound stronger (this also helps to engage the diaphragm). Put a different consonant sound at the beginning of each one:
Too, toe, taw, tah, tay, tee
Soo, soe, saw, sah, say, see
Koo, koe, kaw, kah, kay, kee...etc.

Siren-ing

You can try 'siren-ing'. Make a humming noise and explore the whole range of your voice. Go up and down the scale like a siren. Keep going up and down, up and down, from the lowest note to the highest. Try this again on an 'ng' sound. Mouth open, back of the tongue in an 'ng' sound. Then again on a 'brrrr' sound, with your lips together and vibrating.

If your jaw is tense, you will not usually be able to reach as high or low with the 'brrrr' sound. If your jaw is tense, the 'brrrr' sound will stop unintentionally. This can happen when you are nervous, so is a good way to test whether your jaw is tense.

If it is tense, you can do this exercise: clasp your hands together in front of your chest as if you are praying and with your mouth open and relaxed. Now vigorously move your hands out and away from your chest and back again. Let the sound out, and your jaw should loosen. Now try the siren-ing on the 'brrr' sound again. Is it easier?

Communication techniques

The following approaches are informed by the techniques described by neurolinguistic programming (NLP). NLP was developed by Richard Bandler and John Grinder in the 1970s (Bandler & Grinder, 1981) as a framework for understanding how information and communication is processed by the mind and its application in psychotherapeutic approaches, particularly around self-improvement. Since the 1970s, NLP ideas have been developed and marketed to a wide variety of audiences, particularly in the business world, but have also been taken up by some healthcare practitioners.

Although there are a variety of techniques that have been developed within the range of published works and taught courses relating to NLP, we will focus on basic techniques that will help build rapport as those most appropriate in the CASC and everyday practice.

Rapport is a qualitative aspect of a relationship in which those concerned understand each other's feelings and ideas, and communicate well. In the context of the CASC, rapport is so often talked about as something you developed 'well' or 'not so well' by those who give you feedback. We often comment in our assessments of people who come to see us in clinical practice – 'Good rapport developed'. If rapport is critical, how do you develop it? The rest of this chapter describes techniques for developing rapport.

Developing an awareness of another person's communication style and process

We all have our own communication style and it is important to develop an ability to become aware rapidly of someone else's particular style when you first meet them, especially in the time-limited context of a CASC station. A style will be made of a set of coordinated facial expressions, hand gestures, changes in vocal qualities and bodily postures that are linked to someone's emotional state or a particular thought process. 'Body language' and 'non-verbal communication' are phrases commonly used to describe this.

> **Examples**
> When someone is thinking an idea through in their mind – they may sit still, with a hand rubbing their chin and their eyes turned upward, avoiding gaze.
> When someone is preoccupied and feeling sad – they may drop their shoulder, become still and look at the floor, be very still or fidgety.

Using your peripheral vision to notice the subtle visual aspects of communication is invaluable and again should be practised. These signs include subtle changes in facial expression, eye movement, limb movements and respiration rate.

There is a danger that you could develop a 'painting by numbers' approach to 'reading' body language or non-verbal communication: for example, they are looking down, so therefore the person is sad. Remember that non-verbal communication needs to be understood in the person's unique individual context, i.e. the nature of the situation they are in, their understanding of why you are talking to them as well as their underlying personality traits.

Calibration

Calibration is the process of becoming consciously aware of how someone is communicating both verbally and non-verbally. This conscious awareness requires you to be receptive; when you first start practising these techniques, you cannot be caught up in your own thoughts. Instead, you need to be fully present and observing closely. Using your peripheral vision to notice 'minimal' cues is invaluable. Minimal cues include subtle changes in facial expression, eye movement, limb movements and respiration rate. As such it can be useful to practise this in less-pressured situations at first, perhaps when observing communication between peers. This is likely to be easier than in a patient interview or practice CASC scenario, where you might be constantly distracted by the thought of your next question/diagnostic features/how much time you have left. With practice you can then introduce this increased awareness of other people's communication methods into those situations where you are actively participating and where it will be of most use to you. One particularly useful exercise is to record a practice scenario and watch it back with the sound turned off. Watch for subtle changes in body language and facial expression, and think about what might be being communicated by these. You may be surprised by how much more is going on than you first noticed.

Pacing

Pacing is the next step on from calibration. It is a conscious noting, moment by moment, of the nature and patterns of someone else's communication style and then adjusting your style to better fit with theirs. This is not about simply being aware of the content of the communication but rather the process of it. So when somebody asks you a question, you not only answer the question but also answer the way in which they asked the question. This is a natural, unconscious process most of the time. You 'fall into step' with someone when walking alongside them. One must make this a conscious process in order to take it further and use it strategically.

Matching

Part of pacing someone's communication style is the process of 'matching' – an essential technique in building up rapport with people. This is a technique used intuitively by good communicators. It is also often unconsciously performed among people who know each other well. For it to work effectively it must be done subtly, such that the person with you is not consciously aware of what you are doing. Matching involves using the same communication process(es) that the other person is using, such as body posturing. This is not to be confused with mirroring – which is the process of copying the gestures or movements of another as if you were them in a mirror. This can become very obvious and have a negative effect on rapport. To avoid this and confusing yourself, just think about the idea of approximately matching someone's communication to create a more comfortable, flexible approach.

Body movements

The participant should adopt a similar stance or posture to the other person but this is not simply a case of mimicking them. If a person changes their posture, do not simply copy the same movement immediately. This will come across as awkward and unnatural; also, patients with psychosis might misinterpret this in a paranoid way, which will hamper rapport. Instead, one might notice this and perform a similar movement a short time later.

You might only wish to match one part of a person's posture. Perhaps the hand movements they perform. You might wish to use another part of your body to match what you have observed. Crossed arms could be matched with crossed ankles for example. Sometimes people use their hands to symbolically place ideas, concepts or people in the space around them. You may notice patterns in how people do this, and you could match these.

Breathing

Using your peripheral awareness it is possible to notice someone's breathing rate and pattern. If you can match this subtly, it becomes a powerful and unconscious rapport builder. It also gives you great insight into a person's inner state, such as their level of anxiety or motor retardation.

Phrases and words

We all have our own phrases and frequently used words. When you adopt a patient's phraseology, discreetly this can help develop rapport – and make the other person feel that you are 'speaking the same language'. Be careful with idiosyncratic, slang or peculiar words though; matching these can seem fake unless done after a good rapport has already been developed.

People will often use words that reflect a predisposition to a particular sensory modality, i.e. visual, auditory or kinaesthetic (touch and somatic sensations). You will recognise these patterns easily now that you are aware of them; for example: 'I see your point of view' (visual); 'I hear what you are saying' (auditory); 'I feel I know what you mean' (kinaesthetic). If you notice that someone is frequently using phrases or words within a particular modality, then reflect this in your own language. You should also try to become aware of which modality (if any) you yourself tend to use.

If a person uses a particular phrase or word to describe a property or dimension of their experience, then pace their experience by using it. Such properties might be the strength or size of a sensation or memory. As an example, someone might describe a 'great' feeling of sadness and you should reflect this in the language you use when asking questions – 'When did this great feeling of sadness start?' It may also allow you to explore the problem by establishing differences – 'Do you always feel such a great sadness, or are there times when you can feel lighter (kinaesthetic) or brighter (visual)?'

This is not simply a process of active listening: it is a process of using what you hear to deepen rapport with a person.

Vocal matching

With practice, if you can match the content of somebody's speech, then you can also match the qualities of their speech, i.e. their tone, intensity, tempo and volume. This takes practice and it starts with learning to use your own voice, which is why we would encourage you to do the vocal warm-up exercises (pp. 4–5).

If someone's voice is at one extreme, perhaps whispering or shouting, then completely matching it would not be helpful. You may wish to move yours some way towards it. If someone is whispering, then softening and lowering your voice to a degree will help to build rapport.

Adaptation for difficult dynamics with patients

If a patient is highly anxious or angry, matching their experiences with body language or vocal qualities is unlikely to be helpful and may look a bit ridiculous. You should learn to calibrate their experience quickly through the observations of their verbal and non-verbal communication.

Taking the example of a person who is highly anxious, you may wish to start by slightly increasing the rate of your speech or by making quicker hand movements to match the anxiety-related behaviour of the person. This has to be done with skill and should only be tried when you are comfortable using the basic techniques mentioned earlier in a variety of less-polarised situations. Subtlety is the key and in order to get this, practice developing a precise control over your vocal qualities and a conscious awareness of your body movements.

A further sophistication is to reflect a person's mental state in the language you use. This is not simply a case of using the word 'anxious' or telling the person they look stressed. However, you might use the word 'stress'. For example: 'I would like to stress to you that we are going to do all we can...'. What this technique requires is some preparatory study playing with language to work out which words and phrase work well. As with all of these techniques, making them work is largely about using them appropriately in the moment and adapting them rapidly to do so.

Leading

As you build up your finesse with these skills, you may try matching in one modality of non-verbal or verbal communication while 'anti-pacing' in another modality. Anti-pacing means deliberately not falling into step with somebody's mode of communication. Taking the earlier example of a person who is anxious, you might use quick hand movements and 'anxious' words, but the tone and speed of your voice is soft and calming (anti-pacing the person's own tone and speed of voice). Owing to people's tendency to fall into step with each other, as you develop rapport you can increase the anti-pacing actions and hopefully the person will be led by you into a more relaxed state. At this juncture you could try sitting down if the patient has been standing up to that point. If your rapport building has been good enough, then they may sit down. In a non-CASC interaction this can take as long as it needs to. In the exam you need to get to this point of 'leading' a patient as quickly as possible.

Example
You enter a mock station and find a patient's relative who is very agitated. The scenario suggests that they may be feeling angry as their son has been detained under the Mental Health Act 1983. You note their body language: they are pacing the room when you enter, they stop and place their hands on their hips, they gesture with forceful, quick movements that move towards your personal space, making the scenario feel confrontational. They are speaking at a loud volume and the pitch is more variable than a usual conversational style. Their sentences are either short bursts or longer statements that reference a number of issues in quick succession.

Imagine how you might respond to this in your non-verbal communication. You could match the person's stance, using arm and hand gestures that are animated but are not as forceful or as rapid and are kept out of the personal space of the other person. In terms of your speech, a consistent tone and pitch would anti-pace the other person's communication, but your sentences could pace the person's communication by being kept short and to one discussion point. If they are voicing a multitude of concerns or complaints, focusing on one discussion point can begin to lead the conversation into a more productive exchange.

If you notice that the person's body language changes and their tone and pitch of voice begins to even out, their gestures become slower and are kept closer to the body, their sentences become longer (often as their breathing rate decreases), then you might be able to ask whether they wish to sit down (they may do this naturally).

Practice this 'leading' of people with those you develop rapport with easily (and those in less extreme mental states) to gain confidence in doing it. Focusing on one modality of communication at a time can be helpful. Try to build up to leading with both non-verbal and verbal communication techniques where you can as you progress through this book.

Breaking rapport

There may be times when you do not wish to establish close rapport or need to reduce rapport that has already been established, for example when a patient with manic symptoms is becoming sexually inappropriate. To do this, applying the principles in reverse is effective – i.e. establishing a different vocal quality, language or body posture will help to break rapport or prevent it from forming or limit it.

An everyday example of this is bumping into a friend when you are in a hurry but they are obviously keen to talk. Think about how you adapt your body posture in this situation and how you change your tone of voice and what you might say. Commonly, people keep a greater distance between them, angle their body away from the other person in the direction they want to go, and increase the speed of their speech, giving it a breathless quality – thus conveying that they are in a rush.

Summary

The techniques of calibration, pacing and leading can be seen to be on a spectrum of increasing assertive influence within any interaction – with calibration being a passive stance of observation, pacing being a more active process of adjusting your own communication style and leading being a highly active approach to influencing the communication between you.

Rapidly building an awareness of someone else's communication style and continuously adjusting your own communication style to match it are the first two important steps. When rapport is established, you can try to adjust your communication style and lead the person into a different interaction, and perhaps a different emotional state. As an interaction needs to end, so you can break rapport through again adjusting your communication style.

Underlying all of this is a need to develop an awareness of your own communication style and learning to explore and control the full range of it.

As we have previously mentioned, these techniques are often used unconsciously in talking to those we know well; becoming aware of them might feel uncomfortable and using them more strategically may feel awkward at first. Keep trying them and the process will become much more natural.

Try running through mock stations 1–3 (pp. 49–52) to practice the communication techniques that are described in this chapter.

Reference

Bandler R, Grinder J (1981) *Frogs into Princes: Neuro Linguistic Programming*. Real People Press.
Howell WS (1982) *The Empathic Communicator*. Wadsworth Publishing Company.

CHAPTER 2

Verbal communication skills

The techniques in this chapter focus on gathering information and beginning to manage the flow of a scenario.

Unless you feel very confident, to develop the following techniques try practising them one at a time during an interaction – ideally the next time you see a patient in your clinical practice. You may well overuse them at times and find that the flow of the conversation becomes too broken up. Once through this stage you will get to a point of using them appropriately without overdoing it. By the time you get to the exam you should be blending them together to create a flowing conversational style, which you can maintain despite any distractions, derailment or frank confrontation by the patient. In this chapter we will cover the following verbal communication techniques:

- open/opening and closed/closing questions
- clustering
- signposting
- summarising
- helicoptering
- reflecting
- normalising experiences
- using and bouncing.

Question types

Open/opening questions

An open question is one to which there might be a great variety of responses. 'What happened to bring you into hospital?' is an open question. Starting with an open question has many advantages. It allows the patient to start with what they may find important or most upsetting. It facilitates the building of rapport as you can begin to gather useful information through the variety of responses they might give. With this in mind, it is generally a good idea to start with an open question.

The disadvantage of open questioning is the potential for you to gain irrelevant information (i.e. not relevant to the task at hand in the exam station) or for the patient to become side-tracked. So continuing to use open questions has its down sides. If you are not getting the information you need, you may need to rethink your approach.

Closed/closing questions

When you want to hone in on particular details of what a patient is telling you, you may wish to 'close' the questioning. A closed question is one that limits the potential responses from the patient. This allows you to gain specific information and therefore to be more certain of what is going on for your patient. As an example, you might start a mental state examination by asking 'Have you experienced anything unusual recently?' This is a very open question and could provide a variety of responses. 'Have you ever heard voices that other people can't hear?' is a question that closes down the number of potential responses to the subject of voice hallucinations. The 'ever' is emphasised, keeping the question slightly open as it asks the person not just about the current time but also the past. Compare this with the question 'Are you hearing voices now?' The responses to this question are on some level going either to be 'yes' or 'no', making it a closed question. If the answer is 'yes', you could move back up 'the question tree' and ask 'Can you tell me about the voices?' – a question that is closed to the subject of the voices but open as to the nature of the details you are looking for. These questions could be considered closing questions as you are closing in on the details but at least one element is still open.

Moving up and down the question tree

The skill to develop is to be able to move up and down the question tree from wide, open questions, to closing questions and ultimately to very closed questions. It is the moving up and down in terms of openness that can add to the flow and sophistication of an interaction. You should not always just be moving down the tree consistently from open to closed, nor just jumping from the extremes of very open questions to very closed questions and back again.

As with the examples given, the nature of a question can be closed in one aspect and open in another and it is this combining of elements that allows you to adapt your questions to get what you want without sounding like an interrogator. The simple addition of the word 'ever' or 'now' can transform the openness of a question. These words relate to time. There are of course other words that can relate to spatial parameters, such as 'where' and 'here', which can also alter the openness of a question.

As discussed in the previous chapter, observe yourself in everyday practice and when practising scenarios. What mix of questions do you ask? Are you always asking closed questions and how does this affect your interaction with the patient? What happens if you only ask very open questions? Can you use more closing questions that have both open and closed elements? Watching or listening to recordings of yourself can be really useful here.

There are situations where patients are chaotic in their thoughts and actions, or completely withdrawn and respond little to your questions. In both cases maintaining a line of open questions could be both fruitless and frustrating as the person's thought disorder carries you away to talking about jelly babies or elicits no useful response from an almost mute patient. In this case, controlling the openness of your questions will be key. For a patient with mania, narrowing the questions down to ones with inherently limited responses may help gain control and, more importantly, get specific information that might help you manage the situation. Similarly, closed questions to someone who is barely talking might help you begin to find out some information that sheds light on what they are experiencing and allows you to do something that might alleviate the problem. Consider how difficult it could be for someone who is very distressed and/or withdrawn to answer a completely open question; non-threatening, closed questions can be very useful to help such a person begin to speak. It also presents them with the opportunity to communicate without speaking by nodding or shaking their head.

As we shall see, in the CASC exam using time effectively is essential and one way of doing this is to keep your question style adaptable to the amount of time you have. A closed question is likely to result in a one-second answer, 'yes' or 'no', and that may be all you need or want when trying to cover a few areas in the last minutes of a station. Be careful not to lose the rapport. A way to prevent this is to acknowledge the lack of time, for example 'As we only have a few minutes left, I would like to ask you some specific questions just to make sure I haven't missed anything'. Remember to keep the tone of your voice light and open; you are being warm and empathic even when trying to clarify some key points.

Tip
Avoid initially asking questions using 'Why', as these can be particularly difficult for people to answer. First explore experiences through 'How', 'What', 'When' and 'Where' questions instead, for example: 'How did you feel when that happened?' or 'What was going on when you were feeling like that?'

Specific verbal communication techniques

Clustering

Clustering is a specific questioning technique whereby once a patient gives you an important piece of information, all of the relevant features are explored before moving on. For example, someone mentions that they are experiencing auditory hallucinations; you then proceed to ask about the qualities of those experiences (does the voice talk to them or about them, does it tell them what to do, etc.) before moving on to another aspect of the mental state, which in this case might logically be visual hallucinations (however, the requirements of the station may demand you move on to something a little less directly related). This skill can signpost to the examiner that you follow a clear schema and are structured and methodical in your approach to the history. Clustering can of course happen at different levels; clustering the mental state questions together will sound professional and efficient before you move on to, for example, the social history, which again you can cluster.

There is a danger that you might get side-tracked by the revelation of a symptom or piece of history. The examiners want you to show that you can fully elicit the qualities of a symptom but also hold to the task of the station. So remember to cluster but then move on to the next element of the history.

You may use this technique already in your everyday practice without thinking about it. However, in the exam there is every chance that, owing to the pressure of the situation and the nature of the scenario, this may be forgotten. Hence it is a good idea to start practising the technique in mock situations and become aware of what you are doing in order to hone your skills. Then in the exam you will be likely to use it to maximum effect.

Signposting

Signposting is highlighting that you will be asking or wanting to talk about a particular issue later on in the conversation or acknowledging that you will now be asking about a particular topic. This helps the person you are talking with to follow the conversation and also anticipate what is to come. An example of this would be: 'I would like to ask you more about your sleep in a few moments, but I just want to finish talking about your appetite first: have you been feeling like eating less over the past few weeks?' It might be that you have noticed a particular comment that has been made, recognise that it is important and want to 'signpost' that you will talk about it shortly.

Summarising

Summarising involves repeating back information gathered during an interview in a concise and coherent way. In an exam situation, summarising back to the patient the information that you have found out during the course of the scenario has several valuable benefits. The first is to demonstrate to the examiner and the patient that you have actually been listening to what they have been saying. This helps build rapport with the patient through demonstrating your understanding of their experiences. It also helps the examiner to know that you are following what is going on. The second effect is that it gives you a chance to work out what information you have and what is missing. It frequently prompts further questioning of one aspect of the history you have already touched on or highlights areas you have yet to explore.

> **Example**
> 'So Mr Smith, from what you've told me it sounds like things have been very difficult for you for the past 3 months – you've been struggling to get to sleep and waking up early, you don't have much energy and you're finding concentrating difficult. I'm just wondering, how has your appetite been?'

There is a balance to be had between spending time summarising and continuing to gather information. Frequent summarising will look like you are struggling to find direction in the station (which you may well be). Naturally, summarising relies on you actually listening to the patient and not getting distracted by your own internal thoughts/doubts/narrative (e.g. how bad the last station was). Remember the importance of being fully present and observant.

Helicoptering

At times you may be asked a question that seems to come out of the blue, is somewhat confrontational or disrupts the flow of the conversation. In an exam situation these types of interruptions are normally made with the exact purpose of disrupting your flow or challenging you to deal with the situation.

Helicoptering is a technique in which you hover 'above' the question or confrontation in your response. You might acknowledge the question and stress its importance, but for the moment continue with your original line of questioning, and say you will come back to it (if appropriate). The idea is that you do not get caught up in a line of conversation that takes you away from the task at hand. There is a danger that you could feel anxious in this situation, which then affects your ability to focus and the rapport you have developed. Helicoptering enables you to stay in control.

During your practice sessions try working out some phrases that will help you to 'helicopter' and practise using them. These phrases need to be used in combination with non-verbal communication techniques designed to maintain rapport and keep you in control of the situation.

> **Example**
> You are asked to assess a young lady who is using intravenous drugs in the accident and emergency department (A&E). You have been taking a history from her and she appears to be in an agitated state. While asking her about her family she interjects: 'Can I please just have some diazepam now, I can't concentrate on what you're saying'. Using the helicoptering technique you could say the following: 'I can see it's really hard for you at the moment and I'm sorry for that – but for me to help you properly and safely there are a few more questions I need to ask you before we can talk about you having some medication'.

Reflecting

During a psychotherapy session a therapist is likely to comment on the communication between themselves and the person in therapy, to encourage further reflection and understanding. This technique of reflecting back to the patient requires attentiveness, a degree of confidence and relatively quick thinking to work well. However, it can be effective in drawing attention to an important point and in demonstrating to an observer that you are paying attention and are in control.

An example of this might be someone experiencing manic symptoms who comments on how attractive you are. This can be disruptive and completely put you off your flow of questioning and yet it is a highly valuable moment. This person is actively demonstrating manic symptoms and you need to show that you have picked this up. You might not necessarily respond to it in a confrontational and direct way but perhaps, as in a psychotherapy session, use the information in your next question. For example: 'Have you been making comments about how attractive other people are recently?' You might want to make it more obvious that you felt the comment was inappropriate: 'How have people reacted when you've said that to them, have they perhaps felt uncomfortable?' A note of caution here – addressing this directly can come across as combative and the right tone of voice and manner is paramount, hence practising your non-verbal skills is essential to your CASC preparation.

You have to be confident, but once you feel comfortable doing this, there are endless aspects of the consultation that can be reflected on by the clinician and brought 'into the room'. This could be what the person is wearing, their thought pattern or how they are behaving (e.g. perhaps someone who was not keen on shaking hands with you). This technique is also important in a psychotherapeutic context, as it is essentially a comment on a dynamic element of the conversation.

Normalising experiences

This technique involves using the experiences of others to open up areas of enquiry that may be difficult or sensitive areas. An example is: 'Sometimes when people experience low mood, they can feel so bad that they feel like they do not want to live anymore. I wonder whether that is something you have ever felt?' This technique can help to make connections throughout the conversation to different experiences in such a way that by the end they can be seen as linked, and so helping with a shared understanding of what is happening for that person. This can also be used within the scaffold of diagnostic criteria for particular disorders as described later in the book (see 'Using ICD-10 criteria', pp. 21–23).

Using and bouncing

The aforementioned techniques are building blocks, but used in isolation they will sound blunt and unsophisticated. They must be practised in order for you to use them naturally within the flow of a conversation. One simple phrase to keep in mind is 'use and bounce'. If you use one of the techniques, most of the time, it would be appropriate to bounce into a question or a further piece of information that is pertinent to the subject of the conversation. An example would be if a patient asks you a personal question such as 'Do you have these problems with your kids?' You could reply by saying 'Well, I am here to find out how we might help you and your son. You've told me about some of the difficulties he's has been having and I'd really like to ask you a few more questions... particularly, I wonder, has your son ever harmed himself deliberately in any way?' Remember that this needs to be delivered with appropriate rapport-building non-verbal communication; it cannot simply be said as blankly as the words on this page might suggest.

Mock stations 4–6 (pp. 53–56) can be used to practise the techniques outlined in this chapter.

CHAPTER 3

Taking control

In this chapter we will look at specific aspects of the CASC scenario and how different techniques can help you to take control and manage what we believe to be the most difficult aspect of the exam – that you need to perform a specific task in a very limited time period, far shorter than you would in a real-life scenario. This is one of the most frequent criticisms of the exam in that it is not totally reflective of real life. We would argue that although this is certainly the case, the situation does push you to use your communication and cognitive skills to their very best, showing the examiner what you are capable of doing under pressure and with skilled preparation. We hope that the techniques we describe here will help you to do this.

How long is 7 min?

This might sound like an odd question but in terms of preparing for the CASC, getting a sense of how long 7 min and 10 min are is very important. Station instructions give you specific tasks to complete and you need to make sure that you are able to complete all of these tasks in the time you are given. As part of your exam preparation, try repeatedly setting the timer on your telephone/watch to 7 min and start getting used to how long 7 min really is. You should do the same for 10 min (the time you have for a paired station). You can do this while you are engaged in various activities – such as reading, washing up, having a conversation – as well as while practising stations. This may sound very obvious but it is definitely worth doing. It will truly give you a sense of how long 7 min and 10 min really are, how long they feel in different situations and what you can get done in that time. You might be surprised!

The following techniques are designed for you to get the most out of the short time that you have in the exam scenario. They are best practised within the context of a mock station, as it is the real pressure of the clock ticking that will motivate you to use them (also, announcing that you only have a minute to go while assessing someone in A&E could seem a little out of place). The technique of using diagrams and the structure of the ICD-10 that will be discussed in this chapter is also undoubtedly useful in the right circumstances in everyday clinical practice.

Starting the station well

You have 90s before entering the station to read the instructions. Use this time to take in the key points, and to do this more efficiently read the tasks first. This means that when you are reading the information about the patient you already have a framework to put it in; for example, the station task is to perform a relevant cognitive examination, and then you read they have been disinhibited, so it is probably frontal lobe testing the examiners are looking for. Some people make notes at this time and when you are practising this, it is a good idea to jot down some key words that represent the things you need to cover. However, in the exam this is likely to take time and could distract you. Perhaps it is wise to jot down the patient's name, as you should be using it in your opening introduction and it is very easy to forget this important information during the pressure of an exam situation.

Introduce yourself properly and set the scene. Find a way of introducing yourself that you feel confident and comfortable with (e.g. 'Hello, my name is Dr Josie Jenkinson and I am a psychiatrist. I would like to ask you some questions if that is alright?'). Do not waste any time in the first minute. The information given to you in the instructions can be used to get the station going. Asking a question such as 'Tell me why you've come today', although a nice open question, gives the patient a chance to go off on a tangent and risks you losing control. Starting with something more specifically related to the task required gives you a chance to establish control. For example: 'I understand you have some concerns about taking lithium and I have come to talk to you about them. Perhaps you could start by telling me what you are most worried about?' Obviously if the patient still starts talking about something else, then this is a signal to follow this lead to see where it goes. However, this lead may be as much about the process (i.e. the patient's manic state) as it is about the content.

Keeping the station going

In the middle 5 min you will be trying to achieve the bulk of the tasks of the station. This is where it is important to have developed that sense of how long 7 min is. It is inevitable that things will not always go smoothly and at some point you are likely to be derailed either by yourself or by the patient. When this happens it is important to have an array of tools at your fingertips to help you get back on track and to cover ground quickly and professionally. An example of this is being able to cover the full psychiatric history as efficiently as possible.

During your practice, work out the minimum number of questions that you can use to screen elements of a history. For example, what three questions would you ask to cover the most important aspects of a social history? This technique takes preparation in the run-up to the exam. Spend some time going through a psychiatric history, reducing the number of questions you need to cover each of the sections to the barest minimum that still gives the patient the opportunity to highlight significant elements.

Examples

Risk history

Have you ever harmed yourself or had thoughts of harming yourself? Have you ever harmed or had thoughts of harming someone else? Have you ever been harmed or been threatened by someone else?

Medication history

Are you taking any prescribed or over-the-counter medications at the moment? How long for? Have you ever reacted badly to a medication? Have you been on different medication in the past?

Closing the station

As you hear your 1 min reminder, take stock of where you are up to as you can still cover important ground in the remaining time. Have you got most of the task done? What would be the key questions that would demonstrate that you at least understand what is left to do in the task? If you have completed the task, can you briefly demonstrate understanding of any additional related elements? An example of this could be additional elements of risk. Try not to start an entirely new element of a history or explanation in the closing stages. This is likely to look very inconsiderate to the patient. Ideally, you should be able to summarise back to the patient what you have covered in the station, and in the last 10–20 s bring the station to a close professionally – this leaves an excellent last impression with the examiner. If you have not covered a few areas that you would like to have done, then acknowledge them and the fact that you do not have much time left. In most cases it will be appropriate to suggest that you could meet with the person again to talk further. If appropriate, offer the person further information such as a specific leaflet or direct them to a website.

However the station went and whatever point you left it at, thank the patient before you leave. Good manners and courtesy will always make a good impression.

Using ICD-10 criteria

ICD-10 (World Health Organization, 1992) sets out the diagnostic criteria for psychiatric disorders. Part of what you are trying to demonstrate in the CASC is your ability to diagnose such disorders; therefore it seems wise to refer to the criteria when thinking about structuring your performance in certain stations. However, we are not saying that you should simply run through the diagnostic criteria in the station as this will sound detached and mechanical. You need to be subtler than that, and a useful exercise is to look through ICD-10 criteria and practise converting each criterion into a sensitive question you can ask a patient. A very useful consequence of this is that it helps you with your knowledge revision.

When summarising back to the patient during stations, you could highlight the significant points of the history that would match the criteria of a particular diagnosis in the ICD-10. Subtle use of similar wording to the ICD-10 criteria will allude to your knowledge of it. For example, the patient clearly describes early morning wakening, so you could summarise back to the patient by saying 'It sounds like you are waking more than a couple of hours earlier than you normally would' – this highlights that you know the ICD-10 definition of early morning wakening. Another example would be 'Please tell me if I've misunderstood, but from what you've told me, it seems that you've had these problems for at least the past 2 weeks if not for several months' or 'It sounds like these problems have been troubling you for the past 1 week, is that right?' This demonstrates to the examiner that you are aware of the timescales specified for a particular diagnosis and yet avoids an insensitive checklist approach.

Another useful preparatory activity is to go through the main ICD-10 diagnostic criteria and work out phrases that you can use when summarising the information presented to you. You will of course look less than competent if you use these inappropriately, trying to force the information that you have been given into a diagnosis. A 1-week history of low mood cannot suddenly become a 2-month history just because that is the phrase you have prepared.

The technique outlined above is useful in stations primarily focused on history-taking. In stations that require more explanatory structures, the ICD-10 criteria can be used as a framework around which to build these explanations. Again, the process involves taking the language of the ICD-10 and reflecting it in your explanation but maintaining a non-jargon style.

An example of this is a disorder such as attention-deficit hyperactivity disorder (ADHD). You might start off by highlighting the three main problems in ADHD.

Example
If a child has ADHD they can have problems with paying attention. They can have problems with running around a lot and not sitting still, and not doing what they are told. Perhaps we can look at each of these areas in turn and explore any examples you might have of Johnny's behaviour that fit with them, and then we will be able to discuss what help there is for him.

This is just one example of how you can highlight your knowledge of a condition and the diagnostic criteria and use it to introduce structure to the station. It settles your nerves and signposts for everyone in the cubicle where you are going in this station. Yes it is fairly explicit, but do not forget you are doing it while deploying all your rapport-building skills, from tone of voice to body language.

This technique is similar to the use of diagrams in explaining cognitive–behavioural therapy (CBT). It maps out for you, the patient and the examiner what direction you are taking and it establishes that you are able to control these situations yet maintain a conversational style. It goes without saying that you should avoid lecturing the patient or relative, but rather seek to blend the knowledge they already have with the information that you want or need to give them in order that they can make more use of it. Again, this is not just a skill for the CASC but for everyday practice too.

Modelling a model

There is a well-known saying that 'a picture says a thousand words' and this can be equally true in a CASC station. In sessions of psychological therapies such as CBT or cognitive analytic therapy (CAT), it is an inherent part of the therapy to draw or write things down. This process helps the therapist to educate the patient and, following on from that, for the patient to come to a deeper understanding of themselves. The visualisation involved in drawing a diagram helps to bring more abstract thinking into a concrete structure that can be reviewed and rehearsed as a part of the therapy.

If a CASC station requires you to explain a therapy, an elegant solution is to begin to model that therapy within the station. This demonstrates to the examiner not only your skill but also your ability to conduct the therapy itself. If you would use a diagram to explain CBT in a real session, then adapt the same diagram so you can deploy it quickly in the CASC station.

To give you an example, when explaining CBT you can refer to the 'hot cross bun' model (basically a circle divided into four using straight lines, just like a hot cross bun), which links emotions, thoughts, physical feelings and behaviours. In a CASC station you might start by exploring each of these aspects in turn, and as you do so make notes of what the patient is saying. If you make the notes in such a way that you mirror the hot cross bun model, once you have finished gathering the information, it is then simply a case of labelling each of the areas. The hot cross bun model is thus personalised and therefore made more understandable or meaningful to the patient. This is something that needs a lot of practice as it has to be done with speed and confidence in a CASC situation, and requires you to take control of the process. You have to be very mindful of time and if you find that the process is taking too long, then it is best to short-cut to the completed model. Do not lose sight of the fact that you have to sufficiently demonstrate to the examiner that you have an understanding of CBT.

An explanation of CBT requires more than just outlining the hot cross bun model; it also requires the process of therapy, for instance graded exposure or thought-balancing exercises. You will also need to talk about the nature of sessions, including the number of sessions and the importance of homework between them.

In explaining the nature of psychodynamic therapy, diagrams are unlikely to be useful; however, skilfully modelling the psychodynamic approach in your questions or your responses at times would be a highly effective way of demonstrating your ability. This requires you to have some psychodynamic experience and be comfortable with using the approach, but by the time of the exam you should have this experience.

There may be other stations in which using diagrams to explain complex ideas may be the best way to go. As with all the techniques included in this book, if you are going to use diagrams, make sure you are well practised at doing so, and remember to position the diagram so that others in the station can see it. In the exam you may be highly anxious and any diagram you would like to draw needs to be at your fingertips with only minimal thought required. The exam is not the time to try something out for the first time.

Further developing your communication skills

If you would like to develop your communication skills further, then learning about the specific techniques used in particular approaches or models of therapy may be a helpful next step. Learning about these techniques further broadens your range of how you structure your questions and responses to suit a particular interaction or purpose. Those sitting the CASC should get supervised training experience and teaching in CBT prior to sitting the exam and therefore we have not highlighted the specific techniques from this approach (e.g. Socratic questioning) here as they should be included in your preparation for the exam. Three areas are expanded on below.

Motivational interviewing

Acknowledging that at the heart of much of healthcare is a process of change for a person, motivational interviewing is an approach that draws on an individual's motivation to change in a particular circumstance. It is an approach that takes into account the patient's particular strengths alongside a non-judgemental collaborative approach. An accessible article for those unfamiliar with motivational interviewing has been published in the *BMJ* (Rollnick *et al*, 2010).

There are stations in the CASC where using a motivational interviewing technique may be useful in guiding the conversation. An example of this might be someone who needs to reduce their alcohol use or a pregnant lady who is thinking about coming off opiates.

Although it may not be appropriate to use motivational interviewing techniques throughout a station, one or two well-developed questions can help to really move the conversation forwards, and may be useful where you feel you have not yet understood the needs of the person.

Solution-focused therapy

Solution-focused therapy was developed as a goal-directed, collaborative therapy that focuses on a person's internal strengths and competencies as well as external resources for coping and recovery. This may contrast with the problem-focused approach of other therapies. The following are five particular techniques specific to solution-focused therapy that you may find useful.

The miracle question

This poses the idea that things in a person's life could be miraculously different and then asks them what would be different about that. 'Imagine you could wake up tomorrow and feel well again. What would be different? What would you do differently?' This question has to be used sensitively and followed up with further questions about the details of the imagined future.

Scaling questions

Many clinicians use scaling questions (e.g. 'rate your pain out 10') but developing scaling as a way of exploring a person's experiences can be used in a far more sophisticated way to help recognise the differences in those experiences. Scaling also allows the clinician to track progress over time, both retrospectively and prospectively – 'What would have to change for you to feel 7/10 in your mood more of the time than not?'

Exception-seeking questions

Moods, thoughts, relationships and experiences of pain are rarely absolutely stable. Exploring the inevitable variability in experiences is an important way of identifying the strengths and resources that may enable coping and recovery. Using scaling can be helpful in identifying exceptions. 'So on some days you can feel as good as 6/10 in your mood – what is the difference about those days? Do you do anything differently to look after yourself on those days?'

Coping questions

Positively building on scaling and exception-seeking, coping identifies the occasions when a person managed to cope or is coping. Making it to an appointment might be an example of coping, and exploring what enabled a person to attend the appointment might be a starter for identifying resources and strengths.

Problem-free talk

Medical assessments and interviews can often focus on problems (pain, loss of function) and miss many of the strengths and resources that might be available to a person to cope. Problem-free talk moves the conversation to other areas of life (hobbies, interests) that may be easier to talk about for a person struggling to discuss distressing subjects, and in that allows for the identification of exceptions as well as strengths and resources. In terms of the CASC, you might want to use this cautiously, but a concise, tailored question may help to identify something that would otherwise be missed: 'We have talked a lot about the difficulties in your life at the moment – I wonder whether there is something you do that helps you to feel relaxed?'

Family therapy

There are different types of questioning techniques that have been developed over the years by the school of family therapy, including circular, strategic and reflexive. These share many of the same features as those mentioned earlier; that is, exploring experiences, questioning differences and also using imagined situations to explore change in a facilitative way that challenges thought but does not prescribe any particular action, but hopefully encourages it. In family therapy, the attention is on the relationships between members of the family and as such the questions reflect this. Circular questions explore how a person might understand how another family member relates to their behaviour – 'How do you think your mum would feel about your anxiety?' or 'Who worries the most about your anxiety in your family?'

In terms of the CASC, the person you are talking to is likely to have a family and although they are not there, it may be useful to keep them in mind. Again, this perhaps could be done through one question – 'Who in your family is most worried about you?' The answer to this may give valuable information about the individual's support system and family situation.

Summary

The approaches outlined in this chapter are an advanced set of skills that may provide flexibility to your communication skills, meaning that you are less likely to get stuck in a scenario. One strategic, thoughtful question may 'unstick' a situation and allow a conversation to move on, enabling you to complete the task that has been set.

Doing some reading around these approaches as part of your preparation, and where possible speaking to experienced clinicians who use these techniques, would be a useful step for those who already feel comfortable with the basics and want to push themselves further.

Mock stations 7–9 (pp. 57–60) can be used to practise the techniques covered in this chapter.

References

Rollnick S, Butler CC, Kinnersley P, Gregory J, Mash B (2010) Motivational interviewing. *BMJ*, **340**: c1900.

World Health Organization (1992) *The ICD-10 Classification of Mental and Behavioural Disorders: Clinical Descriptions and Diagnostic Guidelines*. WHO.

CHAPTER 4

Structured presentations

So far we have looked at communication and general structural techniques, but there are some stations that require specific structural approaches to achieve good results. In this chapter we will look at some of these stations. This is not exhaustive coverage but we have aimed to provide some examples so that you can more readily appreciate the structure that is required in the other stations you come across.

Having a structured approach to taking a history of a problem and/or presenting it back to a colleague can be extremely useful. There are many different ways of doing this but one example is to use the mnemonic NOTEPAD – Nature of the problem, Onset (how did it start), Timescale (how long has it been going on for), Exacerbating factors, Palliating (relieving) factors, Associated symptoms, Detrimental effects on the person's life. Another mnemonic useful to remember when discussing an acute problem with a senior colleague is SBAR – Situation, Background, Assessment, Recommendations. These are just two examples and you can devise your own preferred mnemonic based on what you think the most important elements of the history are in different scenarios.

The mnemonic approach has the benefit of being a very simple way of helping you recall lots of information while keeping it structured so that you do not lose your focus in front of a potentially intimidating colleague. In developing structural techniques for stations there are important lessons illustrated by this example. The first is to keep it simple. The mnemonic itself has to be easy to learn and remember, so try not to make it too complicated. The second point is that although it needs to be kept simple, it needs to help you present all the information and knowledge you have, thus minimising the chance of missing something out. The third point is that you will have to recall this technique while being under pressure, so practise it. Do not use it if you thought it up the night before the exam. You almost certainly will not remember it.

Specific structured stations

Case discussion with a consultant

There are some scenarios that require you to discuss a case with a consultant 'over the telephone'. In this situation having a clear structure will help you cover all the areas needed and demonstrate a considered and thoughtful approach to your psychiatric practice.

In some ways this is no different to presenting a patient at a ward round. You need to be able to present the major problems in a concise way, highlighting any significant positive and negative findings. You might then wish to use the predisposing/precipitating/perpetuating factors framework to present the relevant historical details. You do not have much time and telling the consultant about the patient's dog may be irrelevant and could waste precious seconds. You may be familiar with this framework as it is a classic way of formulating a case and frequently taught. The use of this technique in the CASC can be seen as an example of how your practice in the exam can be considered no different to your 'real life' practice, despite the artificiality of the exam situation.

Taking this further, remember also the biopsychosocial framework. We would suggest that this is used primarily in outlining your management plan; it will also demonstrate consideration of all aspects of treatment or management that can be offered to a patient. Using this approach you hopefully will not just talk about medication, but also show consideration of psychological therapies (even if it is to say why you think they would not be appropriate) or suggest the patient attends local groups to improve their social network. If you do not already do this in your day-to-day clinical practice, try getting into the habit of presenting your plans in this way to see whether it helps.

Treatment-resistant schizophrenia and clozapine

In this scenario you need to present the details of the case and then show the thought process and consideration one goes through when thinking about starting clozapine. An example structure would be:

1 Confirm diagnosis
2 Consider drug history
3 Consider adherence
4 Counselling of patient
5 Risks that need to be highlighted
6 Pre-treatment investigations
7 Starting regimen
8 Following up blood tests, including levels
9 Other psychosocial interventions.

This is not necessarily the precise structure you might use but it illustrates the logical flow you are trying to demonstrate. Review the information regarding clozapine prescribing and think how it best fits together.

Remember, the CASC should be considered an 'ideal' situation so you can always suggest that you will provide the patient with all the information and see them the next day, even if in reality this is unlikely to be possible.

Approaches to presenting information to patients and carers: chunking and checking

In addition to the verbal skills we discussed in Part 1, 'chunking and checking' is a useful technique when presenting information to a patient or carer. This method involves breaking down in a structured way the information that you are trying to convey into 'bite-sized' amounts. Before moving on to the next bite-sized 'chunk' of information, you 'check' the patient or carer has understood that bit of information, giving them an opportunity to ask clarifying questions.

When explaining a medication to a patient, you might start with a chunk of information about how the medication works; then pause and ask whether they have understood that bit of the information (the precise way that you do this is up to you, so experiment during your practice). The patient or carer might come back with a question or helpfully repeat some of what you have just said. If they ask questions, be careful not to get too side-tracked and use other verbal techniques to manage this (helicoptering, reflecting, etc). Once you have checked their understanding, move on to the next chunk, which might involve explaining the side-effects of medication.

If you examine patient information leaflets, they tend to chunk information into manageable and appropriate parts. Do not learn these as a script, but do use them as a guide in your practice for the exam as to how you might approach 'chunking and checking'. Take every opportunity in your day-to-day clinical practice to develop and refine this technique. It can be used to hand over to colleagues on call as much as with patients and carers.

CHAPTER 5

Physical examination, investigations and cognitive assessment

So far we have covered various aspects of verbal and non-verbal communication as well as structured approaches to stations. Three types of station included in the CASC that can cause a lot of anxiety for candidates are physical examination, interpretation of results and cognitive assessment. Unfortunately, these are often the stations left until last when it comes to revision – but to perform well they should be included right from the start.

Physical examination

Many of you may have done OSCEs (Observed Structured Clinical Examination) at medical school or as part of your postgraduate training. There is little difference between these and the physical examination stations you will encounter in the CASC. You need to be able to complete an appropriate physical examination in a sensitive, efficient and confident manner in a short amount of time. When preparing for these stations, a good way to start is by devising a protocol for each of the systems you might need to examine (e.g. respiratory, cardiovascular, endocrine), with diagrams if you find these helpful. Then practise the instructions you would need to give to a patient in order for them to understand clearly what you need them to do to follow this protocol. Often during their revision people practise the examination itself but not what they will actually say as they go through it, and then find it difficult to find the right words to communicate clearly in the actual exam – this looks clumsy and feels awkward.

Once you have your protocol and instructions clear, practise. Practise again! These examinations should become fluid and natural so that during the exam you can show both competence and confidence. You should try to present the findings of your examination as you go along in lay language so that the patient can understand them. This demonstrates several skills, but perhaps the most important is your ability to convey information using non-technical, jargon-free language and help a patient feel at ease.

PHYSICAL EXAMINATION, INVESTIGATIONS & COGNITIVE ASSESSMENT

Great opportunities to practise these stations are while admitting a patient to a ward when on-call. See whether you can do a specific examination in 5 min, presenting the findings to the patient as you go along. Ask your patients for feedback if you feel it appropriate. Outside of this you can practise on your peers, friends and family, and ask for honest feedback from them on how it felt to be examined. Videoing is extremely useful. Volunteer to be examined by your peers and take careful note of what things feel awkward and what feels reassuring, and try to incorporate this into your own practice. It is easy to forget what a daunting experience it can be to be on the other side of the stethoscope. If you are really nervous, try practising on a soft toy to start with. Unfortunately they cannot give you any feedback (if they do, you are probably not getting enough sleep).

Tips for physical examinations

- Introduce yourself politely.
- Ask whether the patient would like a chaperone.
- Use the alcohol gel beforehand and afterwards.
- Give a brief introduction with an overview of what you are going to do and ask the patient for consent to be examined.
- Remind the patient to let you know if at any time they would like you to stop, if they feel uncomfortable or if they have any pain.
- Do not waste time taking a history – unless the station clearly asks you to do so.
- Be clear, polite and concise in your instructions.
- Always check whether the person has any pain before feeling or moving a joint, etc.
- Be slick and competent with any instruments you have to use – especially the fundoscope and blood pressure machine.[1]
- Explain what you are doing – this is for the patient and the examiner, and will help you to maintain focus and structure.
- Say when you have finished, thank the patient and summarise key findings.
- Outline the relevant investigations you would like to conduct or any extra information you would like to find out.

Systems or problems that could be featured as a station or part of a station include:

- cardiovascular
- respiratory

---

1. Make sure you have had ample practice with these before the exam day, and try using a few different models as they can function slightly differently. If your hospital is attached to a medical school, see whether you can use their clinical examination rooms and equipment, as they will have plenty of equipment, including heads with different retinal pathologies for practising fundoscopy.

- abdominal
- cranial nerves 2,3,4 and 6 – pupils, fundoscopy, eye movements
- cranial nerves 5 and 7–12
- peripheral nervous system
- cerebellar
- thyroid/neck
- effects of alcohol
- drug misuse – heroin addiction
- withdrawal state
- eating disorders
- extrapyramidal side-effects (EPSE) and other drug side-effects.

An excellent book that can take you through most of the standard physical examinations in depth is *McCleod's Clinical Examination* (Douglas et al, 2013). The AIMS (Abnormal and Involuntary Movements Scale) is a useful examination schedule that can be performed to look for side-effects of psychotropic drugs and is freely available online, as well as being reproduced in several core psychiatric textbooks.

It is worthwhile devising your own schedule for the examinations that may be specific to psychiatry. For example, if you were purely examining a patient for signs of heroin addiction, you would want to specifically look for track marks in the many possible injection sites, pupil size, deep vein thrombosis and temperature, as well as undertaking a urinary drugs screen and blood-borne virus test as part of your additional investigations. The time taken to work these out for yourself is well spent as it will help you to revise specific features of psychiatric illness as well as to remember the schedule you end up devising.

Investigations

Another type of station that can come up is the interpreting investigations station. Here you might be given some blood test results or an electrocardiogram (ECG) for example. Remember to focus on the task and take note of the context of the station. Some stations might ask you to communicate results to a colleague (e.g. a medical registrar or your consultant) or you may need to explain results to a patient.

ECG interpretation

This is one of the most common CASC investigation stations. You might not have had to present an ECG formally since you were in foundation year 1, so this just serves as a reminder.

- Set the scene with a brief description of the patient and current problem
- Note the speed at which the ECG was recorded
- Rate

- Rhythm
- Axis
- P waves
- PR interval
- QRS complex morphology
- ST segment
- T waves
- Any other notable anomalies
- Conclusion and implications for further treatment or investigations

The only way to improve your skills is to look at as many ECGs as possible – a very good basic textbook to refresh your memory is *The ECG Made Easy* (Hampton, 2013). Practice in front of colleagues from other specialties if you can, and it is always worth asking any general practice trainees on your local training rotation for help with this.

Cognitive assessment

Cognitive assessment stations are very common in the CASC. Usually you are given a précis of the patient's problems and asked to perform an appropriate cognitive examination. The Mini Mental State Examination (MMSE) may or may not be specified. For example, you may be told that the patient has been complaining of problems with their memory, and that their partner has noticed some impulsivity and personality change.

The MMSE is inherently structured and you need to be able to recall the structure and do the examination in about 5 min. Unsurprisingly this takes some practice. There are two processes here. The first is remembering the exact content of the test and the second is to work out the clear and quick instructions so you do not waste time repeating yourself or confuse your patient. These two processes are the key to developing your structure and are a necessary starting point for other areas of cognitive testing, namely the specific tests for frontal, parietal and temporal lobes, something that causes a lot of candidates concern. A way of combating this anxiety is to develop an in-depth understanding of what cognitive processes these areas of the brain are involved in. An excellent textbook to help you understand this better and structure your examinations accordingly is *Cognitive Assessment for Clinicians* (Hodges, 2007).

For each of these areas, learn the tests available and the precise instructions you need to give. Then it is a case of practising. Ideally you will develop an internal 'menu' of tests that you can call upon during the station, adapting your approach to the scenario and the clinical history given.

In these stations be polite, introduce yourself and explain the reason for wanting to do the test, but try not to spend too much time on this unless your patient is expressing concern or seems reluctant. Try not to get drawn into taking a history unless the task specifies this; however, it is almost always useful and relevant to check whether the person has noticed any problems with their memory or whether they have any particular concerns. Do check whether the person needs anything to help them perform as best they can, such as glasses or a hearing aid, and also check whether they are confident using a pen before you ask them to write or draw anything. Move as quickly into the testing as you can but remember that this might not always be possible or appropriate, and the patient's reactions to your questions should be your guide. Hopefully you will have enough time to complete your testing, summarise your findings and suggest some next steps that you would like to take. If not, remember to use your last minute well and highlight anything further that you would like to do if you had more time.

Now try practising with mock stations 10–12 (pp. 61–62).

References

Douglas G, Nicol F, Robertson C (eds) (2013) *McCleod's Clinical Examination* (13th edn). Churchill Livingstone Elsevier.

Hampton JR (2013) *The ECG Made Easy* (8th edn). Churchill Livingstone Elsevier.

Hodges JR (2007) *Cognitive Assessment for Clinicians* (2nd edn). Oxford University Press.

Part 2

Planning your preparation

CHAPTER 6

Developing the right knowledge

By the time you get to the CASC you will have sat all three written MRCPsych exams, so your knowledge should have become much deeper. For the CASC, you need to have much more practical knowledge at your fingertips, such as what are the steps to assess testamentary capacity or the therapeutic range for lithium levels.

We would suggest that the knowledge revision specifically for your CASC should start at least 4–6 months before the exam if it is to be done properly. You will need time to feel very secure with your level of knowledge so that you are then able to experiment with how you present in and use practice stations. Here are our top tips for developing your knowledge base.

- A useful start is to make an exhaustive list of the conditions you will need to know about for the CASC. Using the ICD-10 as a guide is useful, but remember there may be conditions which are not in there (e.g. re-feeding syndrome) that can also come up.
- Once you have your list, for each condition you need to know the main symptoms, diagnostic criteria, prognosis and management. To make sense of the management, try writing the different aspects into a 3 × 3 grid, which splits it up into short, medium and long term, and then again into biological, psychological and social areas. This formulation of the management plan will feed into the structure you develop for presenting information in a station, making it much more manageable, concise and complete.
- For every commonly used drug you need to know doses, titrations, side-effects and contraindications. If the drug requires special monitoring through plasma levels or other blood tests, you need to know these too.
- For every form of therapy you need to understand it enough to be able to explain it.
- Use a variety of sources for your revision (e.g. standard textbooks, evidence reviews, National Institute for Health and Care Excellence (NICE) guidelines, websites, patient information leaflets). We have put together a useful list of resources at the end of the book.

Your revision may well be different to your written paper revision in that you should keep a focus on the practical use of the knowledge you gain. Try to always think how best you might explain something as you read it, or how you would need to phrase a question sensitively and concisely to get a specific piece of information relevant to a condition. It might be easier to say that if you are going to be thoroughly prepared for the CASC, there is no area of psychiatry that you can ignore.

CHAPTER 7

Individual preparation

Start with securing your knowledge base as described in the previous chapter and have a look at the additional resources at the end of this book. Prepare a revision plan at least 4–6 months in advance of the exam date, taking into account any major commitments and on-call patterns. As you will have found out in studying for written exams, it can be very difficult to motivate yourself to do exam preparation after a full day of clinical work. The good thing about the CASC is that there are opportunities during your working day to maximise your preparation through practising your skills and getting colleagues to observe you. Approach as many colleagues as you can, particularly Royal College of Psychiatrists examiners or people who have recently passed the CASC, for their help. If you have not had the opportunity to do a job in one of the subspecialties such as intellectual disability or addictions, consider spending some time with the consultant/registrar working in that specialty or revise with trainees in that subspecialty.

When completing your workplace-based assessment with senior colleagues, push them to give you honest and constructive feedback on how to improve your performance, even if they tell you things you find difficult to hear. At this stage being told you are at a level expected of your grade should not be enough.

Record yourself with a video camera practising stations and watch them back. Look at the 'bad' vocal and motor habits you have such as tapping your foot or saying 'So...' a lot. Try to work on stopping these. Notice what you particularly like about how you communicate and build on this. Reviewing recorded stations also helps with your revision of structured stations (such as cognitive assessments) to help you see where you could have phrased something better or whether you missed anything out.

As we have previously mentioned, avoid learning a script for a station. This is a short-sighted way of approaching the CASC and will inevitably trip you up in the exam when the station evolves slightly differently. Try to develop confidence and competence in dealing with whatever is thrown at you – it is what you do in real life. A consultant does not have a script for a Mental Health Act assessment, so you should not need one in the CASC.

Psychological preparation and coping with anxiety on the day

The experience of preparing and going through any exam is undoubtedly stressful. For some it can be a very difficult period, particular if previous experiences of the CASC or other exams have been negative and bred fears and self-doubt. We know from running a CASC preparation course that worries about anxiety (meta-anxiety) and experiencing anxiety on the day of the CASC are a major concern for candidates. For those whose communication skills and knowledge are good, anxiety affecting their performance seems to the biggest barrier to passing the CASC. A little anxiety improves performance, so finding ways of staying in the right zone is an important part of your preparation.

If you are well prepared, try to ease off on the preparation as you get closer to the exam to give yourself a break. Worrying about your communication skills the day before the exam is counterproductive, as you will only increase your performance anxiety and this will have a negative effect on the excellent communication skills you probably have. Here we will offer some techniques for psychological preparation for the CASC and for managing anxiety on the day. As with any technique, they require practice.

The basics

Although not wishing to patronise, it is important to remind yourself of the basic things that can help us manage stress. Eating a balanced diet with healthy foods in regular meals that promote stable energy levels, regular exercise and a regular routine of sufficient sleep will go a long way to helping you prepare. If you have a regular routine already established, such as going to the gym on a Wednesday or a book club a Thursday, try to stick to it as much as possible, while ensuring you have sufficient time for preparation.

Mindfulness

Currently mindfulness is emerging as a form of meditation that has widespread uses in all aspects of our lives. Mindfulness requires regular, preferably daily practice but can be a powerful way of reducing anxiety and stress, improving your concentration and stamina.

Mindfulness is a great way of managing negative self-talk and promoting the sense of being in the moment with a clear mind that will help you stay focused in a station. It can help with listening and responding to what the patient says rather than getting caught up in any of your own, possibly negative, thoughts about the last station or what you have not yet done in this station. It also promotes your ability to remain self-aware and make those adjustments to your communication style that have been described in Part 1. There are several online mindfulness courses now available, including ones that can be accessed via a smartphone app (e.g. Headspace, www.headspace.com; Be Mindful, www.bemindfulonline.com), and these are worth looking into if you are not able to access training in other ways.

Visualisation/mental imagery rehearsal

Mental rehearsal using visualisation techniques has been used by sports and other professionals both before and during big performance events for years (Weinberg, 2008). When it comes to the CASC, visualisation would include imagining yourself performing as you would want to and would do at your best. Try visualising a particular station and how you would respond to particular difficulties successfully, for example a patient asking a tricky question or being angry.

Visualisations should be as detailed as you can make them and contain other elements such as sounds and bodily feelings. Visualisation should include both seeing yourself performing well as an outside observer, as well as through your own eyes and your own body.

To be effective, visualisations should be rehearsed regularly, perhaps at the same time every day. Visualising first thing in the morning could be particularly useful so that on the day of the exam, positive visualisations readily come to mind.

Mentally rehearsing by visualising what your desired experience of the CASC is will help. You should try to imagine what you would like to feel like – perhaps focused, in a calm state of mind and relaxed in your body? Imagine what you would look like doing a skilful performance in the CASC, visualise yourself sitting with the patient in the scenarios. Hear yourself asking questions and responding to queries. How would you like your voice to sound? Can you see/hear/feel yourself using some of the techniques in this book?

Mock rehearsal

As we have consistently highlighted throughout this book, videoing yourself practising mock stations is an incredibly useful tool. Mock exams are also a vital way of getting a sense of how you will cope in the actual exam under strict time pressures and in a more formal environment. Start with more relaxed preparation in terms of practising with others and work towards a really authentic mock exam experience in which there is an 'examiner' writing notes and times are strictly adhered to as you move from station to station.

Many training rotations will organise mock exams in the run up to the CASC exam. Your local training programme administrator will be able to tell you whether this is the case in your area. Try to get involved in as many of these events as possible, if not as a candidate, then as a facilitator or actor. If your rotation does not already run anything like this, then you could organise something yourself or ask your local higher trainee colleagues – it will help contribute towards their workplace-based assessments in terms of teaching experience.

Try to practice the approach you have decided to take to manage anxiety on the day of the exam during your mock CASC (e.g. any particular routines, visualisations). Remember, a mock exam is a chance to practise and rehearse the experience of the exam as well as the stations.

Managing anxiety on the day

A decent breakfast and getting to the exam location well ahead of time are simple ways of managing your anxiety. If you have taken the time to practise mindfulness during your preparation, then try doing a session in the morning, followed by a mental rehearsal of your performance that you have built up in your preparation. Gentle stretching helps to ease the bodily feelings of tension.

Between stations, feelings of anxiety and worry can sometimes be carried over to the next station. Conversely, a positive feeling after a good station can bounce you into a good start at the next one. It is worth taking 10 s to notice what you are feeling and then let negative feelings go in order to start the next station with a clear mind. Consider having a simple mantra that helps you to refocus after each station, such as 'Every station is a new chance to show how good I am'.

Reference

Weinberg W (2008) Does imagery work? Effects on performance and mental skills. *Journal of Imagery Research in Sport and Physical Activity*, **3**: doi: 10.2202/1932-0191.1025.

CHAPTER 8

Group preparation

We think it is very important that a large part of your CASC preparation takes place with a group of peers who are sitting the exam at the same time as you or with peers who have sat the exam recently. Here are our top ten tips.

1. Size of the group – four people is a good number. This allows for one person to be absent on occasion, leaving enough people to run stations usefully.
2. Ground rules – as you will be aware from your readings of group dynamics, ground rules are important. For a group to be mutually supportive you should be clear on what is expected from all members, such as punctuality, prior preparation, and giving constructive feedback. You all need to feel safe enough to make a fool of yourself. If you do not, perhaps this is not the group for you.
3. Organise and prepare – organise a schedule for covering topics/specialties and plan sessions in advance so you can work around people's other commitments.
4. Membership – try and work with people you get on with, who have complementary experiences or skills in different subspecialties to ensure you can cover everything. You want to consider whether the group members are all at the same level of preparation.
5. Consistency – the group will work best if you are consistent in your sessions. We would suggest weekly sessions in the few months before the exam, and then you may wish to increase the frequency in the last month before the exam.
6. Fun – make it a rewarding experience. Plan to do something relaxing after the session (e.g. sharing a meal, going for a run, going to the pub). Each member could take it in turn to host the group and provide refreshments.
7. Feedback – videoing your stations and watching them back as a group can be useful in giving specific feedback. You could agree a structured way of recording feedback on a sheet. See the example structured feedback sheet on non-verbal communication skills in the Appendix.

In general, be specific but not personal, honest and constructive, and think with the others how you might do something differently rather than simply criticising.

8. Expertise/help – enlist the help of senior clinicians who might be willing to give up their time to do a focused session with you on their area of expertise. Choose carefully; think about people who you want to model, for example get a higher trainee in old age psychiatry to come and observe you doing your cognitive assessment stations and then show you how they would approach the task.
9. Importance of observer – to get the most out of the sessions, take it in turns to be an observer. We reach a greater understanding of our practices by contrasting them with others.
10. Fairness – be willing to practise in areas that other people feel less confident in, even if you are really good at them. Other members will hopefully do the same for you.

CHAPTER 9

The day of the exam

The exam is usually held over several days in a sports stadium located in Sheffield. Unless you live locally, we would advise booking a hotel with easy access to the venue for the night before the CASC. Book as soon as you are sent your exam date to avoid any stress associated with last-minute organisation. Think about your travel arrangements in good time – will you feel like driving? Will it be less stressful to get the train? Personally (J.J.), I decided to drive so that I could make a quick exit after the exam and not be stuck on a train with others who had just done the CASC and end up dissecting each station in detail. But that is because I find that sort of thing very stressful. You might want to have an informal debriefing session afterwards with others who have been through the same experience. Bear in mind that most people who have just done the exam will be focusing on the negatives of their performance. Those who have passed the exam recently may have a more balanced view.

The exam venue is large and noisy when everyone is in full flow as there are several circuits of stations going on simultaneously, with stations separated by screens rather than taking place in separate rooms. There are several periods where you are kept waiting in smaller groups in separate rooms before the exam hall is ready. Once you are in the swing of things, the whole day passes very quickly. Bring something to eat and drink as there will be a break in between the morning and afternoon stations. Everyone will be nervous – some people will keep themselves to themselves, some will come armed with folders and do last-minute cramming, some will cultivate an air of confidence and just try to act normally. Do what feels right for you and makes you feel as calm as possible.

Exam etiquette

Remember that in an exam situation you want to be remembered for your excellent performance and professional manner over and above anything else. The examiner does not have time to get to know you and unfortunately people do make snap judgements on how people dress and present themselves. As such it is worth thinking carefully about the first impressions that you give. We would advise that you introduce yourself by your full name and be appropriately formal. Offer a handshake if it feels appropriate (it will not always). Make sure the examiner can see your candidate number. Try not to be distracted by the examiner writing things down and definitely do not try to see what they are writing. Use alcohol gel before and after any physical examination (this will be provided in an obvious place in the station). When you finish, even if the station has gone badly, smile and thank the examiner and the actor. No matter how badly a station goes, you can always leave the examiner with a positive first and last impression.

After the exam

What are you going to do after you have finished your exams? We would recommend booking a holiday as soon as possible if life allows it.

There is more to life than exams and do not lose sight of that. Keep one eye on what you are going to do after you have finished the exam so that the CASC will just be one hurdle you will inevitably get through one way or another. The exam is a gateway to higher training and it asks the question: 'Are you ready to be a senior clinician in psychiatry?' If you believe that you are, then let it show in your performance. Be confident; be a member of the Royal College of Psychiatrists.

Part 3

Putting skills into practice – mock stations

In this section there are four sessions of three mock stations, which map to four of the chapters in Part 1. Each session contains stations in which the skills of the relevant chapter are an important part of the success of those stations. As the skills are additive and as your practice progresses, you should be able to deploy the relevant skills from all chapters in any station. We would advise that you start practising the stations in the designated order, focusing on the relevant skills from the respective chapter. You might find it useful to read the relevant chapters again before attempting the stations.

CHAPTER 10

Mock session 1: Finding your voice

Station 1

Instructions for candidate

Mrs Adams has been booked into your clinic for an initial assessment. She had asked for the first appointment and has turned up 30 min early. She was referred by her general practitioner (GP) who was worried she might be having a 'nervous breakdown'.

- You should take a history of the presenting complaint.
- You are not required to do a risk assessment.

Instructions for actor

You are very anxious, unable to sit down. You have struggled to see the doctor because of your fear of going outside. You want to leave and get back home but you realise you need help.

You have had this fear of going outside your house for 3 years. You have found it increasingly difficult to lead a normal life and spend more and more time indoors. You have arranged your life so you do not have to go out. For example you speak to your sister in America via Skype; you order your shopping via the internet.

Three years ago your partner died in a car crash. Going anywhere near a moving car is particularly difficult for you and on several occasions you have run back home having gone out.

You have been admitted to hospital before, after collapsing on the high street. You had chest pain but the doctors could not find anything wrong with your heart.

You have not been having flashbacks as you were not involved in the crash that killed your partner. Your sleep is poor and you often find it difficult to go to sleep. Your appetite is fine. You still enjoy reading and watching television but find you cannot do this for too long as your concentration has got worse. Your concentration is often disturbed by thoughts of what might happen to you (e.g. get attacked in your house or burgled).

Prior to 3 years ago you would have said you were a very conscientious person who liked to make sure things were perfect.

The aim of this station is not necessarily for the candidate to get a detailed history but to demonstrate skills at dealing with a highly anxious person. Do not begin to calm down until you feel they have taken steps towards building rapport and empathy in a genuine way. Phrases that you feel are 'stock phrases' will not help you relax. If the candidate tries any relaxation techniques, then go with them. If it is done well, show signs that you are becoming more relaxed.

Station 2

Instructions for candidate

You are asked to assess one of your patients on the psychiatric ward after they have been transferred to the ward from the acute medical hospital. The patient took an overdose and cut themselves while on leave from the ward. She now wants to discharge herself. The nursing staff have suggested that she might need to be placed on Section 5(2) of the Mental health Act 1983).

- Take a history of the recent episode of self-harm.
- Perform an assessment of the ongoing risk.
- Consider whether the patient should be detained.

Instructions for actor

You have been admitted to a psychiatric ward for the past 2 months. In the early weeks on the ward you attempted to harm yourself frequently until you were detained under a section of the Mental Health Act to keep you in hospital against your will. The doctors also increased your mood-stabilising medication. Following this you improved in your mood and remained stable with no further thoughts of self-harm.

The doctors started to give some leave off the ward an hour at a time, which they gradually built up to overnight leave to your mother's house. You were taken off the section of the Mental Health Act. You were allowed home for a whole weekend last week.

While on leave you had an argument with your mother. The argument started with a disagreement about what to watch on television but quickly escalated. You cannot cope with this kind of conflict very well and you felt that it was all your fault and that your mother has never cared for you properly.

While upstairs in your bedroom, you took some tablets and harmed yourself by cutting your forearm with a razor you had hidden in your room for a long time. After you had done this you went downstairs and showed your mother the cuts on your arm, which were bleeding profusely. She took you to A&E.

You were treated in A&E but did not tell them about the tablets you had taken.

You are now back on the psychiatric ward. You do not really want to talk to anyone. You feel tired and want to sleep. You do not make good eye contact and are withdrawn. If asked, you do not have any more thoughts of harming yourself. If the candidate is warm in their manner and appears understanding, you tell them more. Whether you tell the candidate about taking the tablets depends on their communication skills. If you feel they are being genuine, then you may be more likely to tell them.

Prior to this hospital admission you had taken one overdose about 5 years ago. You have had a difficult relationship with your mother, and your father left when you were young. Your mother has had frequent boyfriends who have been drunken and verbally abusive at times to her. Your brother is cold and distant. He has little contact with the rest of the family.

You are not hearing voices or seeing unusual things. Your mood is low.

The aim of this station is to try and get the candidate to demonstrate skills at building rapport and empathy quickly. If you feel they are being genuine in these attempts and not robotic, then you open up more quickly about what has happened.

Station 3

Instructions for candidate

Dr Banner, one of your colleagues, would like to speak to you about the patient you have just assessed. They were on call the night the patient was allowed on leave and are concerned about what happened. They are new to psychiatry, having just started the rotation as a part of their GP training.

- Discuss the case with your colleague, paying particular attention to the risk assessment.

Instructions for actor

You are a junior doctor working at a psychiatric hospital as a part of your training to become a GP. You have been finding the rotation difficult as you are not used to dealing with mentally unwell patients. You are a bit scared of coming to work every day in case you get cornered by one of the patients with mania on the ward. You stay in the nursing office a lot of the time.

Recently you were asked to see a young lady who was taken off a section of the Mental Health Act recently and wanted to go home for the weekend. You saw her at 18.00h on Friday.

The nursing staff were worried about her and wanted her to be seen before she went on leave. You saw her and felt she was fine to go home. She reported that she did not have any thoughts of harming herself and was happy to keep taking her medication over the weekend while away from the hospital. You spoke to her mother, who was on the ward waiting to take her home and she was happy to do so.

When you got into work on Monday after being slightly worried by your decision to let her go home, you find that the patient has cut themselves and taken an overdose. This really upset you and you feel it is your fault.

You feel you should have insisted that she stayed in hospital despite the fact that she said she would be fine.

You do not feel you can trust the patients anymore. You feel they are all out to get you and make trouble for you. You just want to go home and not do any more psychiatry. You do not want to go and speak to your consultant as you feel he will judge you and think you are not strong enough.

You have not had a problem like this in the past and you have usually been top of your class.

You have approached one of the other junior doctors who is looking after the patient and asked whether you can have a chat in the mess. You want to make sure the patient is alright and you are not in trouble. You really want to talk about how you are struggling but you do not feel you are able to do this if the other doctor does not develop good rapport with you.

CHAPTER 11

Mock session 2: Talking techniques

Station 4

Instructions for candidate

You are interviewing Mr Jones, a 22-year-old man detained under Section 136 of the Mental Health Act 1983. He was detained after a member of the public reported him acting bizarrely and appearing extremely agitated and distressed. He is now calm, but still showing some bizarre behaviour and seems to be having hallucinatory experiences.

- Interview Mr Jones with a view to eliciting the underlying psychopathology.
- You are not required to undertake a risk assessment and need only ask about relevant background history necessary to undertake the task.

Instructions for actor

You are Mr Jones, a 22-year-old man. You were detained by the police earlier when a member of the public contacted them as they were worried about your behaviour. At the time this happened you were very distressed and hearing a single male voice telling you 'The time has come'. You are not sure what this means, but have been hearing it frequently recently and recognise it as the same voice each time, although you are not sure whose voice it is. You first heard it 6 months ago and it is getting worse. The voice also tells you to 'Make preparations for a journey. You will know what to do' but is not overtly derogatory or threatening. You believe it but do not feel actively controlled. As a result of this you have packed a bag with belongings that you carry at all times. You are very scared that something bad will happen if you disobey the voice, but are not sure what this would be. You also sometimes feel that comments on the television or radio are signals from the voice, and have packed specific belongings you have seen in television shows as you think they will be necessary for the journey. You are not sure what the source of the voice is but believe it must be some form of higher power.

No one else around you appears to have similar experiences. Your family think you are acting oddly and tell you that you are mistaken or making it up. As a result you have stopped talking to them about your experiences as you feel that it must be a secret mission as they do not seem to understand.

You have no other hallucinations (tactile/gustatory/visual/synaesthesia) and your delusion is very specific (as described earlier).

You have no thoughts or wish to harm yourself or others at present and made no attempts to do so.

You have not been on any medication, have no psychiatric or family history of psychiatric disorder, no history of drug or alcohol misuse and are physically well.

The candidate should enquire about a range of experiences in different sensory modalities and the specific details of hallucinatory/delusional experiences to pass this station and to clarify an in-depth understanding of the psychopathology.

Station 5

This scenario is written assuming the patient is female, but can easily be changed if the actor is male.

Instructions for candidate

Miss Smith has walked into the reception of the hospital unit and she wants to see one of the nurses. She states that she is in love with a nurse on the unit and that they are going to get married. The reception staff have asked you to talk to the patient.

- Assess the woman's mental state.
- Assess the risk she poses.

Instructions for actor

You were recently admitted to a psychiatric ward for 2 months for an episode of depression. You were discharged a few days ago. While you were on the ward you had a key nurse called John and you frequently had little chats with him about how you were doing. As you got better you realised you quite liked John and thought that he quite liked you. This feeling grew but you kept it to yourself because you believed that he would get into trouble if you told anyone that he loved you. You wanted to protect him.

After your discharge you went home and kept thinking about him. You are now convinced that he loves you and you need to see him again. You believe everything will work out now as you are no longer a patient on the ward. However, if things are not going to be alright, you now feel that you are prepared to harm other people to make sure you can be together. You have been fantasising about being John's rescuer, killing all the demons that get in your way.

You have had only one other relationship in the past, which ended when you became too paranoid about what your partner was up to. You thought he was having an affair and threatened to kill the person you suspected.

You were drinking heavily before you were admitted to the ward with depression but you do not think you are an addict. You do not use illegal drugs now but have smoked weed in the past. You have little contact with your family at the moment. You were looked after by your single mum as an only child. Every day you worried when she went out to work that she would not come back. As you got older, sometimes she did not come home for several days.

You have been in trouble with the police before (arrested for possible actual bodily harm) but have not been to prison as you were never charged with an offence. You were drunk and the victim had looked at you as though you were odd.

You have had a drink this morning before coming to the hospital. You have a knife with you in case you have to defend your true love. You want to see John and are not prepared to take 'no' for an answer. Your plan is to take John away with you today. You know that if he refuses to go with you it is just for show and you will be prepared to force him.

You are guarded and repeat that you just want to see him and you know he will want to see you.

Station 6

This scenario is written assuming the nurse is male and the patient is female, but can easily be changed if the actor is female.

Instructions for candidate

After you spoke to Miss Smith, she pulled a knife from her bag in the car park and made threats towards the nurse John who she believes is in love with her. The police were called and she was detained in custody but then released before she was assessed by mental health services. The police have contacted the hospital to inform them. You have been asked to discuss the situation with the nurse.

- Discuss with the nurse what has happened, with particular regard to the potential risk to his safety.

Instructions for actor

You are a nurse on a ward and are aware that one of the patients you looked after caused a bit of a scene recently, but you have been off work and have just come back, so are not sure of what happened. One of the doctors has asked to speak to you.

You live alone in a flat 10 miles from the hospital. You normally cycle to work. Your family lives in Scotland.

You are shocked by what the doctor tells you and very scared. You want to know what they are going to do about it. You keep asking how are they going to keep you safe.

You press the candidate repeatedly if they fail to give you enough information. If they do not know something, then pick up on that and ask what they are going to do about it.

If they are not adequately reassuring, you become more anxious.

CHAPTER 12

Mock session 3: Taking control

Station 7

Instructions for candidate

You have been asked to talk to a patient about CBT after she was interviewed by the consultant, who thinks she would benefit from it for her severe anxiety. The patient would like to know more about what the therapy involves.

- Explain CBT to the patient.

Instructions for actor

You are a patient on a psychiatric ward. You were admitted with thoughts of ending your life after it felt your life had got on top you and you felt very anxious with no chance of getting away from it. You had not being sleeping for several days and had a poor appetite. You were worrying about a lot of things. For a long time you have spent most of your day worrying about things and as a result have been unable to get on with life.

You have had panic attacks in the past and these have been getting more frequent. You feel your heart racing in your chest and you feel breathless. You also feel sweaty. You think you are going to die when this happens. You have to sit down in a quiet place for at least an hour. You have been to hospital twice after such attacks. You have started avoiding the places where you have had panic attacks in the past.

You have thoughts that pop into your head all the time about bad things that might happen. At times you do little rituals, such as tapping your feet five times; this helps you feel less anxious.

You have been on treatment with antidepressants, but would like to find out about CBT as the consultant thinks it will benefit you.

You have concerns that it might make you worse but cannot say why. You want to know what the treatment involves. You want to know whether it will work and if it does, can you stop taking the antidepressants?

Your speech is a little fast and you tend to talk about irrelevant details.

Station 8

This scenario is written for a male actor but can easily be changed if the actor is female.

Instructions for candidate

Amy, who is 15 years old, has recently been assessed by your team and has been diagnosed with anorexia nervosa. Her father would like to talk to you about the condition. He would like further information as he was not at the assessment (Amy's mother was).

- Answer the father's questions about anorexia.

Instructions for actor

You are Amy's father. She has recently been seen by the child and adolescent mental health team and has been diagnosed with anorexia nervosa. Amy's mother was at the initial assessment and she has not been able to tell you much about what the team said about the diagnosis. You telephoned the team and they suggested you came with Amy to have a further chat. Amy did not want to go, so they agreed to see you on your own.

You have noticed over the past year that Amy has been eating very little. She does not eat breakfast and you are not sure what she eats at school. She very rarely joins the family for dinner, and frequently says she has lots of coursework to do and spends a lot of time in her room.

At times you have smelled smoke on her clothes and you are not sure whether she has started smoking. You have also noticed that some of the senna tablets you are taking have gone missing. Senna is a type of laxative you take when you have to take pain medication for your back as it makes you constipated. Your back has always been a problem and periodically becomes very painful with shooting pains down from your bottom to your leg. Amy is your only child. Part of you would still like another but you and your partner have stopped trying and you seem to have lost your desire for it. You are glad in a way that life has settled into a regular pattern.

Although Amy is not eating much and claims to be burdened with coursework, she seems to be doing a lot of dance classes – three times a week now. Even though you are pleased she is looking after herself and you thought she was perhaps a little overweight when she became a teenager, you are now worried that she has lost too much weight. When you try to talk to her about it, she is guarded and often walks off.

She recently collapsed at school and was admitted to the children's ward at the hospital. Following this the doctors there referred her to the child and adolescent mental health team. The doctors on the children's ward said some of the 'salts' in her blood were wrong.

Your partner went with Amy to the appointment for the initial assessment. You told your partner you were busy at work that day. In fact you were having lunch with a colleague who you have been flirting with for the past few months. You are considering having an affair with her but are conflicted by a sense of guilt. Amy's problem is taking over all your lives and you feel you need an escape. You are finding it difficult to talk to your partner for fear they might read your mind.

You have lots of questions about the diagnosis of anorexia nervosa. You have only heard about it in relation to supermodels on the television – making themselves sick to keep themselves thin. You would like to know:

- what has caused the condition – part of you feels it must be your fault. If you feel that the candidate suggests it is your fault as her parent, then you may become angry or tearful
- what the treatment is
- whether Amy will get better.

Station 9

Instructions for candidate

Mr/Mrs Lancaster's son has been referred to the child and adolescent mental health service as his school have concerns about his behaviour. He appears to have difficulty getting on with other children at school.

- Interview his parent and take a relevant history that would enable you to make a probable diagnosis.
- You do not have to discuss the diagnosis with the parent.

Instructions for actor

You are the parent of a child called Tom, who is 5 years old. In the past few months, Tom's school have been increasingly concerned by his behaviour and you have noticed more and more that he is not like other children.

He prefers to play on his own with particular toys. He often gets very upset when he cannot play with these toys or have them with him. He tends to play with them in exactly the same way. He does not really enjoy dressing up and playing cowboys.

He does not play well with other children and does not share his toys. He has been violent at school towards children who have tried to take his toys. He can play for hours with the same toys and you are not worried about his ability to concentrate.

He does not like walking on certain surfaces such as deep pile carpets; he prefers wooden surfaces which he went through a phase of licking when he was playing on them. He has gone through phases of having rituals he has to do, such as walking through a doorway sideways.

His speech has been slow to develop and he does not quite use his words as you would expect. He does not seem to get 'knock-knock' jokes when you tell them. When you tell him off it appears to make little difference. He does not get upset and does not really make eye contact that often.

If you plan to do something or tell him something is going to happen and it does not, he gets quite upset.

He can walk with no problems, and he is up to date with all his immunisations. He has no other medical problems. He was born normally and on time. There is no family history of any conditions that you are aware of but your partner's brother has always been considered a bit odd by the family.

You get on well with your partner and have been enjoying parenthood so far, although it seems to be getting harder as Tom is getting older. You would like to have another baby.

If the candidate asks whether you have any questions, ask them whether they think it is anything serious and whether it will get better.

The features described above are suggestive of autism spectrum disorder.

CHAPTER 13

Mock session 4: Structured stations

Station 10
Instructions for candidate
You have been asked to review the ECG of a patient on the ward who is being treated with clozapine. He started clozapine 4 weeks ago and has been breathless over the past few days. He is not diabetic and has no previous medical history. He was diagnosed with schizophrenia aged 20. The medical student with you would like to know what the ECG means.
- Interpret the ECG and present your findings to the medical student.

Instructions for actor
You know that an ECG shows the electrical activity in the heart and that the different patterns show different things. Your knowledge is vague about what each of the different parts mean. You ask the candidate to talk you through how to interpret an ECG and what this ECG shows.

If you feel they do not explain any aspect well, you ask them to explain again until you are sure you understand it.

Station 11
Instructions for candidate
Miss Jones suffered a head injury 2 years ago. Her family have reported concerns that she is behaving oddly. They gave the example that she appears to be gambling a lot and boasts about having had 100 one-night stands in the past year. You have been asked to assess Miss Jones' cognitive function.
- Perform a focused assessment of the patient's cognitive function.
- You do not have to perform a risk assessment.

Instructions for actor
You are flirtatious and unless the candidate addresses this appropriately you continue to escalate this behaviour. If they address it in an inappropriate

manner, then you can become more hostile and less willing to complete the tasks they set you, asking more questions about what the tasks involve.

You have a concrete understanding of the world. So if the candidate asks you what is meant by a phrase such as 'people in glass houses should not throw stones', you make a literal interpretation of this and say because they will break windows. Make a similar literal interpretation of alternative phrases they may use.

If they ask you to copy a sequence of hand movements then you cannot do this and repeat one movement over and over again.

All other tests they ask you to do you can perform normally to the best of your ability and as long as the instructions are clear.

Station 12

Instructions for candidate

Mrs Smith is a 65-year-old lady who had a stroke 1 month ago. She has made a good recovery but there is concern that there may be some residual cerebellar damage.

- Take a history from and examine Mrs Smith to elicit any signs of cerebellar pathology. Address any concerns she may have.

Instructions for actor

You have recently had a stroke and following this you have noticed you are a bit unsteady on your feet and also have a tremor when performing tasks. You have noticed in particular that when you go to pick up a cup of tea your hand shakes a lot. Your speech is fine and you have noticed no visual disturbance. Otherwise you are well and cooperate with the candidate. You are very anxious about your symptoms and want to know whether they are going to go away or get worse, and whether there is anything you can do about them.

The candidate should ask relevant questions and then proceed to formal examination along the lines of the following:

- dysdiadochokinesis
- ataxia (yes)
- nystagmus
- intention tremor (yes)
- speech (e.g. British constitution)
- heel–shin test (yes).

The candidate should sensitively address your concerns, reassuring you without giving false hope and giving appropriate advice.

Resources

Here are resources that will help in your quest for CASC success.

Alzheimer's Society

A vast array of useful leaflets on all aspects of dementia – including benefits, lasting and enduring power of attorney, and testamentary capacity (www.alzheimers.org.uk/site/scripts/documents_info.php?documentID=160).

Child and adolescent psychiatry

Beat

Useful and up-to-date information on eating disorders (www.b-eat.co.uk).

Young Minds

The charity dedicated to improving the mental health and well-being of children and young people as well as supporting parents and carers. The website provides well-written information sheets for both young people and their families. It is useful to read these for clear explanations of the most common disorders experienced by children and young people (www.youngminds.org.uk).

DVLA (Driver and Vehicle Licensing Agency)

The DVLA website has up-to-date and accurate information about driving with a disability or health condition and taking different psychotropics as well as advice for doctors on what to do about patients who are driving and misusing alcohol or illicit substances (www.dft.gov.uk/dvla/medical/medical_drivers.aspx).

ICD-10

Provides clinical descriptions, diagnostic guidelines, and codes for all mental and behavioural disorders commonly encountered in clinical psychiatry. Available in print and online (www.who.int/classifications/icd/en/).

Mental Health Act 1983: Code of Practice

The *Code of Practice* provides professionals with information on how to carry out their roles and responsibilities under the Mental Health Act 1983, to ensure that all patients receive high-quality and safe care. It is also guides patients, their families and carers on their rights (www.gov.uk/government/uploads/system/uploads/attachment_data/file/396918/Code_of_Practice.pdf).

MIND and Rethink

MIND and Rethink are two excellent large mental health charities that publish a large amount of information regarding mental health problems, which is freely accessible online. Particularly useful for revision are their leaflets on the Mental Health Act 1983 (www.mind.org.uk/information-support/legal-rights/mental-health-act; www.rethink.org/living-with-mental-illness/mental-health-laws/mental-health-act-1983).

National Institute for Health and Care Excellence

Look at the guidelines for major mental health conditions. You should be able to describe stepped care models in lay terms. The guidelines are available on the website or as a downloadable app (www.nice.org.uk).

Royal College of Psychiatrists

The exam pages on the College's website should be your first stop when planning for your CASC. You will find the curriculum here, a guide for candidates as well as example videos of CASC stations (www.rcpsych.ac.uk/traininpsychiatry/examinations/about/mrcpsychcasc.aspx).

The patient information leaflets that are freely available on the College's website are also a wealth of useful tips on how to explain the different aspects of most mental health problems. They are written in simple language and have very useful basic information on incidence, recovery rates and inheritability (www.rcpsych.ac.uk/healthadvice/problemsdisorders.aspx).

The Maudsley Prescribing Guidelines

Ideally, read the latest version from cover to cover, and quote it at all social gatherings. In all seriousness, you need to read it and know it. The Maudsley Prescribing Guidelines are available in print, as an eBook and as an app. Key sections to focus on are: use of psychotropics in pregnancy and in breastfeeding, monitoring regimes (e.g. lithium), and use of clozapine.

Appendix

CORE SKILLS IN THE CASC

Circuits 1 and 2: Non-verbal and verbal communication skills feedback form

Please circle the relevant box for each skill area and make additional comments where possible

	No/little use of skill	Limited use of skill requiring further practice	Uses skill but inconsistently, requiring further practice	Consistent use of skill or technique	Accomplished use of skill or technique	Sophisticated and advanced use of skill or technique
Adaptive vocal qualities (tone, volume, speed, timbre)	No obvious responsive change in vocal qualities. Unempathic vocal qualities	Attempts changes to vocal qualities but not reflective or appropriate to context	Changes to vocal qualities are reflective and appear helpful in building rapport but not maintained	Maintained use of changes to vocal qualities to reflect patient and positive effect on rapport	Clearly able to use changes in vocal qualities with refinement to continued positive effect	Subtle changes in vocal qualities and skilled use of all aspect of vocal qualities to build rapport in difficult contexts
Matching/mirroring	No evidence of changes in body posture or movement in keeping with matching/mirroring	Attempt to matching/mirroring patient with little effect on rapport/empathic stance	Uses matching/mirroring but not maintained throughout, uses occasionally, appears clumsy	Uses matching/mirroring consistently throughout to build rapport in most circumstances	Uses matching/mirroring with sensitivity in more difficult circumstances	Mastery: subtle and sensitive use, appears part of natural style in all circumstances
Pacing to leading (advanced skill)	No evidence that candidate is pacing patient's experience	Cannot be observed to pace but is adapting communication in attempt to do so	Seen to pace patient experience but not maintained	Pacing evident and maintained appropriately – rapport enhanced	Pacing achieved quickly and used well. Evidence of anti-pacing appropriately	Pacing and anti-pacing appear natural. Leading evident in communication

Circuits 1 and 2: Non-verbal and verbal communication skills feedback form (continued)

Please circle the relevant box for each skill area and make additional comments where possible

	No/little use of skill	Limited use of skill requiring further practice	Uses skill but inconsistently, requiring further practice	Consistent use of skill or technique	Accomplished use of skill or technique	Sophisticated and advanced use of skill or technique
Question construction	Closed questions only or poor use of open questions	Starts with open questions but quickly resorts to closed questions	Uses open and occasionally closing questions, resort to closed question where open could be used	Uses open, closing and closed questions appropriately to aid communication and information gathering	Uses all types of questions to aid communication in more difficult situations	Subtle use of question structure to reflect subject and patient context to maximise communication and information
Verbal techniques: clustering/ summarising/ helicoptering/ reflective	None of the verbal techniques used	One or two of the techniques used in a disruptive way. Does not aid communication	Uses techniques pertinently but with clumsy phrasing, abrupt but not disruptive	Uses techniques appropriately in directing flow of conversation	Blends techniques with questions to help maintain flow	Uses techniques in a natural way, blending them into a controlled flow of communication

Additional comments

67

CORE SKILLS IN THE CASC

Circuit 3 – Structured approaches

Please circle the relevant box for each skill area and make additional comments where possible

	No/little use of skill	Limited use of skill requiring further practice	Uses skill but inconsistently, requiring further practice	Consistent use of skill or technique	Accomplished use of skill or technique	Sophisticated and advanced use of skill or technique
Awareness/ management of time	No awareness of time and how to manage it	Recognition of time limits but clumsy response to them with awkward statements	Attempts to respond to time limits with limited success (e.g. unable to finish appropriate closing statements)	Evidently responds to time limits with appropriate opening and closing statements	Good opening statements that quickly get to task, thoughtful closing statements completed	Has good sense of time to inform tempo and focus. Sophisticated opening and closing statements
Knowledge-based structure	Does not use knowledge to inform structure	Uses knowledge in checklist approach to assessment. Lecture style of knowledge giving regardless of patient context	Uses knowledge in an explicit way that is clumsy but attempts to respond to patient contexts both in giving and taking information	Knowledge is incorporated into questions through simple construction. Obvious but not jarring. Knowledge given in a conversational style but remains largely doctor-driven	Knowledge structures are partially informed by the patient's ideas. Uses knowledge structures in a sophisticated way to construct questions	Sophisticated, practised structures used, blends knowledge giving and taking information effectively to enhance patient understanding. Neither patient nor doctor appearing to drive conversation
Overall task focus and control	Does not manage task	Attempts to control task but unable to do so owing to limited skills	Manages to control/ complete task some of the time but struggles if derailed	Able to complete task in most situations with effective use of skills	Combines skills to manage more difficult situations and remain on task	Appears to effortlessly maintain focus on task despite difficulties or distractions

Additional comments

Index

Compiled by Linda English

AIMS (Abnormal and Involuntary Movements Scale) 32
Alzheimer's Society 63
anorexia nervosa 58–59
anti-pacing 9
anxiety
  in candidate 40–42
  in patient 8–9, 26, 49–50
ataxia 62
attention deficit hyperactivity disorder (ADHD) 22
autism spectrum disorder 59–60

biopsychosocial framework 28
blood pressure machine 31
body language 5–6, 9, 10
body movements 7
breathing 7

calibration: communication skill 6
case discussion: with consultant 28
cerebellar pathology 62
child and adolescent psychiatry 22, 59–60, 63
chunking and checking: information to patients/carers 29
circular questions 26
closed/closing questions 13, 14
clozapine 28–29, 61
clustering: verbal communication technique 14–15
cognitive–analytic therapy (CAT) 23
cognitive assessment 20, 33–34, 44, 61–62
Cognitive Assessment for Clinicians 33

cognitive–behavioural therapy (CBT) 23–24, 57
colleagues 39, 41–42, 43–44
communication skills 3, 18, 24–26
  adaptation for difficult dynamics with patients 8–9
  aspects of communication 3–4
  calibration 6
  core 3–11
  developing awareness of another person's communication style 5–8
  leading 9–10
  matching 7–8
  non-verbal 9, 10, 16, 17, 18, 66–67 (Appendix)
  pacing 6–7
  question types 12–14
  rapport breaking 10
  techniques 5
  verbal 10, 12–18, 53–56, 66–67 (Appendix)
  vocal warm-ups 4–5
competence, unconscious 3
coping questions 25
cranial nerves 32

diagnostic criteria: ICD-10 21–23, 37, 63
diagrams 23–24, 30
drug misuse 32
drugs *see* medication
DVLA (Driver and Vehicle Licensing Agency) 63

ECG Made Easy, The 33
electrocardiogram (ECG) interpretation 32–33, 61

69

INDEX

exam
  afterwards 46
  day of 45–46
  etiquette 45–46
exception-seeking questions 25

facial expression 5–6
family therapy 26
feedback 31, 39, 43–44, 66–68 (Appendix)
frontal lobe testing 20, 33
fundoscope 31

group preparation 43–44

hallucinations 13, 14–15, 53–54
hand movements 5–6, 7, 8, 62
heel–shin test 62
helicoptering: verbal communication technique 16
heroin addiction 32
history taking 15, 20–21, 22, 27
'hot cross bun' model 23

ICD-10 diagnostic criteria 21–23, 37, 63
individual preparation 39–42
information
  gathering 12–18
  leaflets 64
  to patients/carers 29, 30, 64
instructions 20
introducing yourself 20, 46
investigations 32–33

jaw tension 5

knowledge development 37–38

leading: communication skill 9–10, 66 (Appendix)

McCleod's Clinical Examination 32
mania 10, 14, 17, 20
matching: communication skill 7–8, 66 (Appendix)
Maudsley Prescribing Guidelines 64

medication 37
  clozapine 28–29, 61
  history 21
  Maudsley Prescribing Guidelines 64
  side-effects 32
Mental Health Act 1983 51
  Code of Practice 64
  Section 5(2) 50
  Section 136 53
mental imagery rehearsal 41
meta-anxiety 40
MIND 64
mindfulness 40–41
minimal cues 6
Mini Mental State Examination (MMSE) 33
miracle question 25
mirroring 7, 66 (Appendix)
mnemonic approach 27
mock rehearsal 41–42
mock stations 19, 47–62
  finding your voice 49–52
  structured stations 61–62
  taking control 57–60
  talking techniques 53–56
modelling therapy 23–24
motivational interviewing 24

neurolinguistic programming (NLP) 5
NICE (National Institute for Health and Care Excellence) 64
non-verbal communication 5–6, 8
  skills 9, 10, 16, 17, 18, 66–67 (Appendix)
normalising experiences: verbal communication technique 17
note making 20
NOTEPAD mnemonic 27

open/opening questions 12–14
OSCEs (Observed Structured Clinical Examination) 30

pacing: communication skill 6–7, 66 (Appendix)
parietal lobe testing 33
patients
  anxiety 8–9, 26, 49–50
  closed questions 14
  communication skills and 5–10
  feedback 31

INDEX

information for 29, 30, 64
name of 20
thanking 21
person-centred approach vii
phraseology 7–8
physical examination 30–32
predisposing/precipitating/
 perpetuating factors framework 28
preparation planning 37–46
 exam day 45–46
 group 43–44
 individual 39–42
 knowledge development 37–38
problem-free talk 25–26
psychiatric disorders: knowledge
 development 37
psychiatric history 20–21
psychodynamic therapy 24
psychological preparation 40–42
psychosis 7
psychotherapy 5, 16–17, 23–26, 28, 57
psychotropic drugs *see* medication
pumpkin face/raisin face: vocal
 warm-up 4

questions 20, 67 (Appendix)
 circular question 26
 closed/closing questions 13, 14
 clustering 14
 coping questions 25
 exception-seeking questions 25
 family therapy 26
 from patient 16, 29
 history taking 15, 21
 ICD-10 criteria 22
 miracle question 25
 moving up/down question tree 13–14
 open/opening questions 12–14
 question words 14
 scaling questions 25
 types 12–14

rapport 5–10, 14, 15, 51, 52
recordings 6, 14, 31, 39
re-feeding syndrome 37
reflecting: verbal communication
 technique 16–17
rehearsal
 mental imagery 41
 mock 41–42
relaxation techniques 50

resources 63–64
Rethink 64
risk assessment 50, 51, 54–56
risk history 21
Royal College of Psychiatrists 39, 46, 64

sadness 8
SBAR mnemonic 27
scaling questions 25
schizophrenia
 clozapine 28–29, 61
 treatment-resistance 28–29
scripts, learning viii
self-harm 50–52
sensory modality: words 8
sexually inappropriate behaviour 10,
 61–62
signposting: verbal communication
 technique 15
siren-ing: vocal warm-up 4–5
social history 21
Socratic questioning 24
solution-focused therapy 25–26
stations
 closing 21
 keep it going 20–21
 mock 19, 47–62
 paired 19
 starting well 20
 structured 27–29, 39, 61–62, 68
 (Appendix)
stress 40–42
structured presentations 27–29, 39,
 61–62, 68 (Appendix)
subspecialties 39, 43
summarising: verbal communication
 technique 15–16, 21, 22

taking control 19–26, 57–60
temporal lobe testing 33
therapy modelling 23–24
'third umpire' viii, 4
thought disorder 14
time management 19–26, 68 (Appendix)
travel arrangements 45
treatment-resistant schizophrenia:
 clozapine 28–29
tremor, intention 62

using and bouncing: verbal
 communication technique 17–18

INDEX

verbal communication skills 10, 12–18
    feedback form 66–67 (Appendix)
    question types 12–14
    techniques 14–18, 53–56
videoing 31, 39, 43
visualisation: mental rehearsal 41
voice 14, 66 (Appendix)
    consultation voice 4
    mock session 1 49–52

vocal matching 8
vocal warm-ups 4–5
see also hallucinations
vowel punching: vocal warm-up 4

wakening, early morning 22
words 7–8, 13